Spanish for Emergency Medical Services

Breanne Blot

Copyright © 2020 Breanne Blot All rights reserved

The characters and events portrayed in this book are fictitious. Any similarity to real persons, living or dead, is coincidental and not intended by the author.

No part of this book may be reproduced, or stored in a retrieval system, or transmitted in any form or by any means, electronic, mechanical, photocopying, recording, or otherwise, without express written permission of the publisher.

ISBN-13: 9798553435547
ISBN-10: 9798553435547

Cover design by: Art Painter
Library of Congress Control Number: 2018675309
Printed in the United States of America

Contents

Introduction	5
Part 1: Spanish Language Basics	8
Part 2: Greetings & Commonly Used Language	64
Part 3: Assessment & Intervention	81
Part 4: Vocabualry	118
Part 5: Dispatch	163
Closing Comments	179

This book is dedicated to those who make a difference everyday.
For those who have lost their lives by serving others,
and those who sacrifice so that others may live.
This book is dedicated to all first responders and their families.

Introduction

Communication is a fundamental part of being a first responder. As we know, it can mean the difference between running a good or bad call. Many different aspects go into human communication, but for the purpose of this book, we will focus on how to quickly and effectively communicate in the Spanish language. The goal of this book is to provide you— the first responder or medical professional— with the appropriate knowledge base of Spanish in a way that is both manageable and relevant to the field of emergency medicine.

Dialectal Disclaimer

It should be noted that there are many different dialects within Spanish. Some words or phrases may be different from what you already know. In order to remain consistent, this book will include language that is most common to Spanish speakers from Mexico.

Explanation of Layout and How to Best Utilize This Book

This book is perfect for complete beginners and intermediate Spanish speakers alike. *Part*

1: Spanish Language Basics and *Part 2: Greetings & Commonly Used Language* are specifically designed for complete beginners and those who need to brush up on some of the language basics. The first two sections build a strong foundation that will help you excel as you advance into the later sections and continue your education beyond this book. Parts 3-5 teach you relevant questions, responses, and vocabulary that are specifically used by paramedics, EMTs, dispatchers, and other medical professionals. *Part 3: Assessment & Intervention* includes patient assessment questions and common responses, as well as other practical language. *Part 4: Vocabulary* provides an extensive list of vocabulary that is organized by topics relevant to the field of EMS, including: cardiology, trauma, medical, and more. *Part 5: Dispatch* has commonly used questions and responses that will be most useful for dispatchers.

A quick note before you get started:

Throughout this book, there are two different forms of the word "you" that will be used interchangeably. There is an informal way to address people which is known as the "**tú**" form, and there is a formal way to address people which is the "**usted**" form. Depending on who you are addressing, either the "tú" or "usted" form will be more appropriate. The "**tú**" form is more often used in informal settings with friends. On the other hand, the "usted" form is more often used in formal settings when meeting someone for the first time or when there is an inherent hierarchy. You will see both forms used throughout the book but take note that you can change the use of "you" based on the context.

Part 1: Spanish Language Basics

It is extremely useful to know the linguistic basics of Spanish, including: the alphabet, grammar, and some of the basic communication words. Learning the basics first will boost your ability to communicate once you reach the more advanced sections. Part 1: Spanish Language Basics section includes: the alphabet, pronunciation, grammar, numbers, and practice examples.

PRONUNCIATION

This book includes a "phonetic pronunciation" section alongside every Spanish word and phrase to help with the pronunciation process. The purpose of this is to help develop your pronunciation skills so that you can pronounce words using the correct phonemes (sounds) that are used in Spanish. This will help develop your accent and accelerate your ability to communicate.

Let's start off with the alphabet, then some explanations of special cases and sounds.

The Spanish Alphabet

Letter	Spanish Pronunciation	English Pronunciation	Phonetic Sample from English
a	a	ah	awesome
b	be	beh	bend
c	ce	se	send
d	de	deh	den
e	e	eh	enter
f	efe	eh-feh	fiction
g	ge	heh	happy and girl
h	hache	ah-che	'h' is silent in Spanish
i	e	ee	even
j	jota	ho-tah	hello
k	ka	kah	kayak
l	ele	eh-leh	love
m	eme	eh-meh	million
n	ene	eh-neh	never
ñ	eñe	eh-nyeh	canyon
o	o	oh	over
p	pe	peh	pen
q	cu	ku	car
r	erre	er-reh	river
s	ese	eh-seh	silver
t	te	teh	ten
u	u	oo	zoo
v	uve	oo- beh	ben
w	doble ve	doh-bleh-beh	winter
x	equis	eh-kees	sixth
y	ye	yeh	yesterday
z	zeta	ze-tah	buzz

It's important to note a couple of things about some of the letters above. As you may have realized, most of the letters are quite similar to English in the way they are pronounced. However, there are a couple of letters that change pronunciation depending on their location. It is imperative that you know these differences.

The letter "C"

When 'C' comes before 'H' it is pronounced like the English 'ch' in chin.

Spanish examples: chancla *n.* (sandel), champña *n.* (champagne).

The letter "G"

When "g" comes before the vowels **a, o,** and **u**, it's pronounced like the English 'g' in *great*.
Spanish examples: garantizar *v.* (to guarantee), guerra *n.* (war), gol *n.* (goal).

When "g" comes before **i** or **e**, it's pronounced like the English 'h' in *hello*.
Spanish Examples: gigante *adj.* (giant), gente *n.* (people).

The letter "L"

When there is one 'l' in a word, it is pronounced as the English 'l' in *ligament*.
Spanish examples: Literalmente *adv.* (literally), lotería *n.* (lottery).

Words with a double 'l' are pronounced as the English 'y' in *yesterday.*
Spanish examples: llamar *v.* (to call), calle *n.* (street).

The double "r" -- 'rr'
When there is a singular 'r' in a sentence, it is pronounced like the English 'r' in river.
Spanish examples: río n. (river), sangre *n.* (blood).

When there is a double "r" in a word, it is pronounced as a trill.
Spanish examples: carro *n.* (car), correr *v.* (to run).

The letter "X"
'X' is generally pronounced as 'ks' like in the English word *kicks.* However it can also be pronounced as the English raspy *h, s* or even *sh* sounds.
Spanish examples:
'Ks': examen *n.* (test)

'H': México *n.* (Mexico)
'Sh': Xicalango *n.* (is a small town in Mexico)

A note on accents:

á, é, í, ó, ú, ü, ñ

In Spanish, accents are used to differentiate words. Accents on letters imply that there is a rise in intonation when spoken, and constitute a different meaning in the written form.
For example: si (if) vs. sí (yes), mas (but) vs. más (more), año (year) vs. ano (anus).

GRAMMAR

This section will include basic information about Spanish grammar. Once mastered, it can help accelerate your knowledge of Spanish by building from what you already know. This section includes: Adjectives & Adverbs, Plurals, Gender & Articles, To be, Demonstratives, Personal Pronouns, Possessives, Prepositions, Questions, and Verb Conjugation.

ADJECTIVES & ADVERBS *Describing People or Things/ Doing Things*

Adjectives generally come after the noun of a sentence in Spanish. On the other hand, adjectives come *before* the noun in English. For example, in the sentence *"the cute dog",* the adjective (cute) comes before the noun (dog).

Examples:

    El perro grande [el perr-ro gran-deh] (The large dog)

    La mujer bonita [la mu-hair bo-nee-tah] (The beautiful woman)

The endings change depending on singularity or plurality and gender— which will be covered next.

Adverbs are adjectives that describe an action - for example, she runs *quickly*. The suffix "-ly" in English is very common among adverbs. *Literal* is an adjective and *literally* is its adverbial form. In Spanish, this same adverbial suffix is shown as "*-mente*".

Examples:
    Rápido [rá pee doh] (quick) becomes **rápidamente** [rá pee dah mente] (quickly)
    Fácil [fá-seel] (easy) becomes **fácilmente** [fá seel mente] (easily)
    Lento(a) [len-toh] (slow) becomes **lentamente** [len-ta-mente] (slowly)

PLURALS, GENDER & ARTICLES *Naming People/Things*

Nouns in Spanish have a "gender" which can either be *masculine* or *feminine*. Every noun generally has articles in front of it, that mean "the" or "a/an". The articles that pertain to each noun depends on its gender and plurality. The articles for masculine nouns are: **el, los, un, unos**. The articles for feminine nouns are: **la, las, una, unas.**

The articles and noun-endings change depending on its gender and plurality. Masuline nouns have their corresponding articles (el, los, un, unos) and end in **"-o"(for singular)** and **"-os"(for plural)**. Likewise, feminine nouns have their corresponding articles (la, las, una,unas) and end in **"-a" (for singular)** and **"-as" (for plural).** It's important to know that some words, particularly those ending in consonants, have **"-es"** as their ending in the plural form. For example, *las ciudades* [las see-oo-dad-es] (the cities) and *los hospitales* [los os-pee-tal-es] (the hospitals) have an "-es" plural ending.

Let's take a look at some examples of masculine and feminine nouns and their corresponding articles.

Definite Articles *(English equivalent to 'the')*

Masculine + Singular	el	(The hospital) el hospital [el os-pee-tal]
Masculine + Plural	los	(The hospitals) los hospitales [los os-pee-tales]
Femenine + Singular	la	(The ambulance) la ambulancia [la ambu-lan-sia]
Femenine + Plural	las	(The ambulances) las ambulancias [las ambu-lan-sias]

Indefinite Articles *(English equivalent to 'a')*

Masculine + Singular	un	(An arm) un brazo [un bra-zo]
Masculine + Plural	unos	(Some arms) unos brazos [unos bra-zos]
Femenine + Singular	una	(A leg) una pierna [una pee-er-na]
Femenine + Plural	unas	(Some legs) unas piernas [unas pee-er-nas]

PERSONAL PRONOUNS

The personal pronouns in Spanish are as follows:

I	Yo	We	Nosotros (as)
You	Tú	You all	Vosotros (as)
He/ She/ You formal / It	Él/ Ella/ Usted	They/ You plural.	Ellos Ellas Ustedes

There are a couple of important things to note when it comes to personal pronouns. *Usted* is the formal form of *you* that is used when talking to strangers or someone of status or importance. Remember to use *usted* to address teachers, bosses, and anyone with high status. Next, make note of best how to use nosotros (we). The ending of *nosotros* changes depending on who you are describing. When addressing a group of strictly men *or* a group of men and women, use *nosotros* with the "-os" ending because that is the most appropriate form for that context. When addressing a group of strictly females, use *nosotras* with the "-as" ending, as that is the most appropriate from. Take note that *vosotros* (you all) has the same gender rules as *usted*. Vosotros is used strictly in Spain, so the more commonly used form of "you all" is *ustedes.*

TO BE Describing People/Things - *ser vs. estar*

There are two equivalent forms of the English verb 'to be' in Spanish. **Ser** and **Estar** are two verbs with the same meaning that change depending on context. Knowing these differences will facilitate the communication process. A good rule of thumb to use when deciding between *ser* and *estar* is the following statement:

"How you feel or where you are, always use the verb *estar.*"

Feelings and location indicate the use of the "to be" form *estar*. Descriptions and characteristics indicate the use of the "to be" from *ser*.

Ser (to be)

Ser is used to describe lasting attributes. Use *ser* when you are talking about someone or something with permanent characteristics. Use the acronym "DOCTOR" to remember when to use *ser*.

D- Descriptions: Ella es fuerte [eya es fu-er- teh] (She is strong)

O- Occupation: Soy paramédico [soy un para- médi-koh] (I am a paramedic)

C- Characteristics: Eres inteligente [er-es in-teli- hen-teh] (You are intelligent)

T- Time/date: Son las doce [son las do-say] (It's twelve o'clock)

O- Origins: Somos de Los Estados Unidos [so-mos de los esta-dos uni-dos] (We are from the United States)

R- Relationship: Él es mi pareja [él es me par-eh-ha] (He is my partner)

Yo soy	*I am*	Nosotros (as) somos	*We are*
Tú eres	*You are (informal)*	Vosotros (as) sois	*You all are*
Él/ Ella/ Usted es	*He/She is You are (formal)*	Ellos/ Ellas/ Ustedes son	*They/ you all are*

Estar (to be)

Estar is used to describe temporary states of being and location. Use the acronym "PLACE" to remember when to use *estar*.

P- Position: Ella está en el edificio [eya está en el ed-ee-fee-see-o] (She is in the building)

L- Location: La medicina está en la ambulancia [la meh-ee-seen-ah está en la ambu-lan-see-ah] (The medicine is in the ambulance)

A- Action: Estoy manejando [es-toy mon-eh-hand-o] (I am driving)

C- Condition: Ellos están enfermos [eyos est-án en-fer-mos] (They are sick)

E- Emotion: La paramédica está feliz [la para-méh-dee-ka esta fe-lees] (The paramedic is happy)

Yo estoy	I am	Nosotros (as) estamos (as)	We are
Tú estás	You are	Vosotros (as) estáis	You all are
Él/ Ella/ Usted está	He/She is You are (formal)	Ellos/ Ellas/ Ustedes están	They/ you all are

DEMONSTRATIVES *Giving Instructions/ Indicating Location/ Pointing Things Out*

Demonstratives are used to point out an object or person in relation to the speaker. English demonstratives are: here, there, this, that, these, and *those*. In Spanish, demonstratives change depending on their gender and plurality.

Singular	Masculine	Femenine	Plural	Masculine	Fememnine
this	**este**	**esta**	these	**estos**	**estas**
that	**ese**	**esa**	those	**esos**	**esas**
that (way over there)	**aquel**	**aquella**	Those (way over there)	**aquellos**	**aquellas**

Examples:

    Este paciente [es-te pasi-en-teh] (This patient)

    Estos pacientes [es-tos pasi-en-tehs] (These patients)

Esta persona [es-ta per-sona] (This person)
Estas personas [es-tas per-sonas] (These people)

Ese hombre [ese om-breh] (That man)
Esos hombres [esos om-brehs] (Those men)

Esa mujer [esa mu-hair] (That woman)
Esas mujeres [esas mu-hair-es] (Those women)

Aquel libro [ak-el lee-bro] (That book over there)
Aquellos libros [ak-ey-os lee-bros] (Those books over there)

Aquella persona [ak-eya per-sona] (That person over there)
Aquellas personas [ak-eyas per-sonas] (Those people over there)

POSSESSIVE ADJECTIVES Possessing

Possessive adjectives help determine to whom something belongs. There are different ways to format possessive adjectives. This next section will cover short-form and long-form adjectives.

Short-form

Short-form possessive adjectives are the most common way to express possession and change based on the gender and plurality of the noun. In this case, the possessive adjectives go in front of nouns. Let's take a look at their forms and some examples.

	Masculine Singular Form	Masucline Plural Form	Femenine Singular Form	Fememinine Plural Form
(I) Yo	mi	mis	mi	mis
(You) Tú	tu	tus	tu	tus
(He/She) Él/ Ella	su	sus	su	sus
(You formal.**) Usted**	su	sus	su	sus
(Us) Nosotros	nuestro	nuestros	nuestra	nuestras
(You all) Vosotros	vuestro	vuestros	vuestra	vuestras
(Them) Ellos/ Ellas	su	sus	su	sus
(You all/ They) Ustedes	su	sus	su	sus

From the chart above, you can see that the most notable changes are between the *nosotros* and *vosotros* forms. These possessive adjectives adapt to the gender *and* plurality of the noun. On the other hand, all other possessive adjectives only adapt to plurality and *do not* factor the gender of the noun. Remember that short-form possessive adjectives go before the noun in a sentence. Let's look at some examples.

Examples of short-form possessive adjectives:

Mi coche [me ko-cheh] (my car)
Mis coches [mes ko-chehs] (my cars)

Tu casa [to ka-sa] (Your house)
Tus casas [tos ka-sas] (Your houses)

Su perro [su peh-rroh] (His/Her dog)
Sus perros [sus peh-rros] (Their dogs)

Nuestro gato [nue-stro ga-toh] (Our cat)
Nuestros gatos [nue-stros ga-tohs] (Our cats)

Nuestra casa [nue-stra ka-sa] (Our house)
Nuestras casas [nue-stras ka-sas] (Our houses)

Vuestra silla [vue-stra sya] (Your chair)
Vuestras sillas [vue-stras syas] (Your chairs)

Vuestro libro [vue-stro lee-bro] (Your book)
Vuestros libros [vue-stros lee-bros] (Your books)

Long-form

Spanish uses long-form possessive adjectives to emphasize the owner of something, a relationship, or to contrast one owner with another. Long-form possessive adjectives must match the noun they modify by corresponding to its gender and plurality. Long-form possessive adjectives go after the noun in a sentence.

	Masc. Singular Form	Masc. Plural Form	Fem. Singular Form	Fem. Plural Form
Yo	mío	míos	mía	mías
Tú	tuyo	tuyos	tuya	tuyas
Él/Ella	suyo	suyos	suya	suyas
Usted	suyo	suyos	suya	suyas
Nosot-ros	nuestro	nuestros	nuestra	nuestras
Vosot-ros	vuestro	vuestros	vuestra	vuestras
Ellos/Ellas/Ud.	suyo	suyos	suya	suyas
Uds.	suyo	suyos	suya	suyas

Examples:

El gato es **mío**. [el ga-toh es mío] (The cat is mine.)
Los zapatos son **tuyos**. [los zapa-tohs son tu-yos] (The shoes are yours.)
La taza es **suya**. [la ta-za es su-yah] (The mug is yours. (*formal*))
La ambulancia es **nuestra**. [la ambu-lan-sia es nue-stra] (The ambulance is ours.)
Los coches son **vuestros**. [los ko-ches son vue-stros] (The cars are ours.)
Los coches son **suyos**. [los ko-ches son su-yos] (The cars are yours.)

PREPOSITIONS *Giving Instructions/ Indicating Location/ Pointing Things Out*

Prepositions are used to locate things in time or space. Below are some of the most common prepositions in Spanish.

English	Spanish
to, at	a
before, in the presence of	ante
under	bajo
with	con
against	contra
of, from	de
from, since	desde
behind	detrás (de)
in, on, at	en
between, among	entre
until, toward	hacia
until, toward	hasta
for, in order to	para
for, by	por
according to	según
without	sin
about, on, upon, above, over, around	sobre
after, behind	tras

Examples:
> **Vamos al hospital** [ba-mos al os-pit-al] (We're going to the hospital)
> **La medicina está en el armario** [la medi-seen-ah está en el ar-mar-io] (The medicine is in the cabinet.)
> **¿Dónde está su bolsa?** [dón-de está su bol-sah] (Where is your purse?)
> **Está debajo de la mesa** [está de-baho de la mesa] (It's below the table.)

QUESTIONS *Asking Questions/ Negating*

Question words are an essential part of language. This section includes a chart with some of the most common question words with a couple of practice examples.

English	Spanish
Who?	¿Quién?
What?	¿Qué?
When?	¿Cuándo?
Where?	¿Dónde?
Why?	¿Por qué?
How, what?	¿Cómo?
Which?	¿Cuál?
Which ones?	¿Cuáles?
How much?	¿Cuánto?
How many?	¿Cuántos?
From where?	¿De dónde?
Why, for what?	¿Para qué?
To where?	¿Adónde?
To whom?	¿A quién?
Where/ whereabouts?	¿Por dónde?
With whom?	¿Con quién?

¿De dónde eres? [de dón-de eh-res] (Where are you from?)
¿Con quién vive usted? [kon key-en bee-beh oo-sted] (With whom do you live?)
¿Dónde está la medicina? [dón-de está la meh-deei-seen-ah] (Where is the medicine?)
¿Cómo se siente? [kó-mo seh see-en-teh] (How do you feel?)
¿Qué pasó? [keh pa-só] (What happened?)
¿Cuántas personas hay aquí? [kwán-tas per-sonas ay a-kee] (How many people are here?)
¿Cuándo empezó el dolor? [kwán-do empe-zó el doh-lor] (When did the pain start?)

VERB CONJUGATION

Verb conjugation is an essential part of forming coherent sentences. Spanish conjugates verbs by having an infinitive form in which there is a root and ending. The infinitive form is the unconjugated form of the verb. The root of the word remains the same (most of the time) and the ending changes based on temporal tense and to whom or what the verb is conjugated.

Spanish has three different types of verb endings. Verbs either end in, **-ar, -er,** or **-ir**. Each set of verbs have their corresponding verb endings. For this first part we will look at the verb endings for the present tense.

-AR Endings (present tense)

Yo *I*	**o**	Nosotros (as) *We*	**amos**
Tú *You*	**as**	Vosotros (as) *You all*	**áis**
Él/ Ella/ Usted *He/ She/ You formal/ It*	**a**	Ellos Ellas Ustedes *They/you all*	**an**

For "-ar verbs", remove the "-ar" ending of the verb and add the corresponding ending to the root of the word. Here are some "-ar" verb example sentences.

Hablar (to talk)
   Yo hablo [yo ah-bloh] (I talk)
   Tú hablas [too ah-blahs] (You talk)
   Él/Ella/Usted habla [el/eya/oo-sted ah-blah] (He/She/It talks)
   Nosotros hablamos [nos-oh-tros ab-la-mos] (We work)
   Vosotros habláis [vos-oh-tros ah-bla-ees] (You all talk)

Ustedes/Ellos/Ellas hablan [oo-sted-es/eyos/eyas ah-blan] (They talk)

Notice from the examples above that the root of the verb stayed the same (habl-) and the "-ar" ending was removed and replaced with the appropriate corresponding ending. The root of the word retains its meaning and the ending changes to match the subject.

-ER Endings (present tense)

| Yo
I	**o**	Nosotros (as) *We*	**emos**
Tú
You	**es**	Vosotros (as) *You all*	**éis**
Él/ Ella/ Usted
He/ She/ You formal / It	**e**	Ellos/Ellas/ Ustedes *They/you all*	**en**

Here are some "-er" verbs and example sentences.

Correr (to run)
Yo corro [yo korr-ro] (I run)
Tú corres [too korr-res] (You run)
Usted/Él/Ella corre [eya korr-reh] (He/She/It runs)

Nosotros corremos [nos-oh-tros] (We run)
Vosotros coméis [bos-oh-tros kom-éh-ees] (You all eat)
Ustedes/Ellos/Ellas corren [oo-sted-es/eyos/eyas korr-ren] (They run)

Again, the root of the verb stayed the same and retained its meaning while the ending of the verb changed to create its desired meaning.

-IR Endings (present tense)

Yo *I*	**o**	Nosotros (as) *We*	**imos**
Tú *You*	**es**	Vosotros (as) *You all*	**is**
Él/ Ella/ Usted *He/ She/ You formal / It*	**e**	Ellos/Ellas Ustedes *They/you all*	**en**

Vivir (to live)
Yo vivo [yo bee-bo] (I live)
Tú vives [too bee-bes] (You live)
Usted/Él/Ella vive [el bee-beh] (He/She/It lives)
Nosotros vivimos [no-so-tros bee-be-mos] (We live)

Vosotros vivís [bo-so-tros bee-bees] (You all live)

Ustedes/Ellos/Ellas viven [oos-ted-es es-cree-ben] (They live)

Included in this next section are some of the most commonly used regular verbs. Regular verbs follow the normal rules for verb conjugation, which means that to conjugate correctly, all you must do is remove the ending from the root of the verb and replace it with the appropriate ending (based on temporal tense and to whom the verb is being conjugated).

Ayudar *(to help)*

Yo *I*	**ayudo**	Nosotros (as) *We*	**ayudamos**
Tú *You*	**ayudas**	Vosotros (as) *You all*	**ayudáis**
Él, Ella, Usted *He/ She/ You formal / It*	**ayuda**	Ellos/ Ellas/ Ustedes *They/you all*	**ayudan**

Comer *(to eat)*

Yo *I*	**como**	Nosotros (as)	**comemos**
Tú *You*	**comes**	Vosotros (as) *You all*	**coméis**
Él, Ella, Usted *He/ She/ You formal / It*	**come**	Ellos/ Ellas/ Ustedes *They/you all*	**comen**

Cortar *(to cut)*

Yo *I*	**corto**	Nosotros (as) *We*	**cortamos**
Tú *You*	**cortas**	Vosotros (as) *You all*	**cortáis**
Él, Ella, Usted *He/ She/ You formal / It*	**corta**	Ellos/ Ellas/ Ustedes *They/you all*	**cortan**

Escuchar *(to listen)*

Yo *I*	escucho	Nosotros (as) *We*	escuchamos
Tú *You*	escuchas	Vosotros (as) *You all*	escucháis
Él, Ella, Usted *He/ She/ You formal / It*	escucha	Ellos/ Ellas/ Ustedes *They/you all*	escuchan

Fumar *(to smoke)*

Yo *I*	fumo	Nosotros (as) *We*	fumamos
Tú *You*	fumas	Vosotros (as) *You all*	fumáis
Él, Ella, Usted *He/ She/ You formal / It*	fuma	Ellos/ Ellas/ Ustedes *They/you all*	fuman

Tomar *(to drink,* also *to take)*

Yo *I*	**tomo**	Nosotros (as) *We*	**tomamos**
Tú *You*	**tomas**	Vosotros (as) *You all*	**tomáis**
Él, Ella, Usted *He/ She/ You formal/ It*	**toma**	Ellos/ Ellas/ Ustedes *They/you all*	**toman**

IRREGULAR VERBS

While there are hundreds of irregular verbs in Spanish that each have their own unique set of rules, we will cover irregular verbs that are most commonly used in everyday communication. It's important to have awareness of irregular verbs so that you know how to correctly conjugate them as you increase your Spanish lexicon. Irregular verbs do not follow the same conjugation rules as normal verbs, and have a unique set of conjugations. Below are some of the most common irregular verbs. *Ser* and *estar* are included as Spanish irregulars and have their own section listed above.

Tener *(to have)*

Yo *I*	**tengo**	Nosotros (as) *We*	**tenemos**
Tú *You*	**tienes**	Vosotros (as) *You all*	**tenéis**
Él, Ella, Usted *He/ She/ You formal / It*	**tiene**	Ellos/ Ellas/ Ustedes *They/you all*	**tienen**

Poder *(to be able to)*

Yo *I*	**puedo**	Nosotros (as) *We*	**podemos**
Tú *You*	**puedes**	Vosotros (as) *You all*	**podéis**
Él, Ella, Usted *He/ She/ You formal / It*	**puede**	Ellos/ Ellas/ Ustedes *They/you all*	**pueden**

Poner *(to put)*

Yo	pongo	Nosotros (as) We	ponemos
Tú *You*	pones	Vosotros (as) *You all*	ponéis
Él, Ella, Usted *He/ She/ You formal / It*	pone	Ellos/ Ellas/ Ustedes *They/you all*	ponen

Decir *(to say)*

Yo *I*	digo	Nosotros (as) We	decimos
Tú *You*	dices	Vosotros (as) *You all*	decís
Él, Ella, Usted *He/ She/ You formal / It*	dice	Ellos/ Ellas/ Ustedes *They/you all*	dicen

Ver *(to see)*

Yo *I*	**veo**	Nosotros (as) *We*	**vemos**
Tú *You*	**ves**	Vosotros (as) *You all*	**veis**
Él, Ella, Usted *He/ She/ You formal / It*	**ve**	Ellos/ Ellas/ Ustedes *They/you all*	**ven**

Querer *(to want)*

Yo	**quiero**	Nosotros (as)	**queremos**
Tú *You*	**quieres**	Vosotros (as) *You all*	**queréis**
Él, Ella, Usted *He/ She/ You formal / It*	**quiere**	Ellos/ Ellas/ Ustedes *They/you all*	**quieren**

Saber *(to know facts)*

Yo *I*	**sé**	Nosotros (as) *We*	**sabemos**
Tú *You*	**sabes**	Vosotros (as) *You all*	**sabéis**
Él, Ella, Usted *He/ She/ You formal/ It*	**sabe**	Ellos/ Ellas/ Ustedes *They/you all*	**saben**

Dar *(to give)*

Yo *I*	**doy**	Nosotros (as) *We*	**damos**
Tú *You*	**das**	Vosotros (as) *You all*	**dais**
Él, Ella, Usted *He/ She/ You formal/ It*	**da**	Ellos/ Ellas/ Ustedes *They/you all*	**dan**

Seguir *(to follow)*

Yo *I*	**sigo**	Nosotros (as) *We*	**seguimos**
Tú *You*	**sigues**	Vosotros (as) *You all*	**seguís**
Él, Ella, Usted *He/ She/ You forma/ It*	**sigue**	Ellos/ Ellas/ Ustedes *They/you all*	**siguen**

REFLEXIVE VERBS

Finally, it is important to have knowledge of reflexive verbs. You can recognize reflexive verbs by the reflexive pronoun "se" at the end of the infinitive form. They are used when a person performs an action to or for himself/herself. For example, **bañar<u>se</u>, llamar<u>se</u>, ir<u>se</u>**, and many more. Essentially, reflexive verbs are used when the subject and direct object of the sentence are the same entity.

To conjugate a reflexive verb, the reflexive pronoun comes off the end of the verb and is placed in front of the verb. The remaining -ar/-er/-ir verb is then conjugated to the desired person or object and tense. Since reflexives are used when the subject and direct object in the sentence are the same, the reflexive pronoun will always correspond with the verb conjugation.

Listed below are the reflexive pronouns. Remember that each pronoun will always correspond to its verb.

Yo / I	**me**	Nosotros (as) We	**nos**
Tú You	**te**	Vosotros (as) You all	**os**
Él, Ella, Usted He/ She/ You formal / It	**se**	Ellos/ Ellas/ Ustedes They/you all	**se**

Here are some of the most commonly used reflexive verbs and their conjugations.

Acordarse *(to remember)*

Yo / I	**me acuerdo**	Nosotros (as) We	**nos acordamos**
Tú You	**te acuerdas**	Vosotros (as) You all	**os acordáis**
Él, Ella, Usted He/ She/ You formal / It	**se acuerda**	Ellos/ Ellas/ Ustedes They/you all	**se acuerdan**

Irse *(to leave)*

Yo / I	**me voy**	Nosotros (as) We	**nos vamos**
Tú You	**te vas**	Vosotros (as) You all	**os vais**
Él, Ella, Usted He/ She/ You formal / It	**se va**	Ellos/ Ellas/ Ustedes You all/They	**se van**

Ponerse *(to put on)*

Yo *I*	**me pongo**	Nosotros (as) *We*	**nos ponemos**
Tú *you*	**te pones**	Vosotros (as) *You all*	**os ponéis**
Él, Ella, Usted *He/ She/ You formal / It*	**se pone**	Ellos/ Ellas/ Ustedes *You all/They*	**se ponen**

Sentirse *(to feel)*

Yo *I*	**me siento**	Nosotros (as) *We*	**nos sentimos**
Tú *you*	**te sientes**	Vosotros (as) *You all*	**os sentís**
Él, Ella, Usted *He/ She/ You formal / It*	**se siente**	Ellos/ Ellas/ Ustedes *You all/They*	**se sienten**

As you can see in the tables above, the reflexive pronoun "se" is removed from the end of the verb and placed in front. The reflexive pronoun corresponds to the subject (i.e. who is completing the action).

To finish up on reflexive verbs, here are some examples used in sentences.

My name is Alexander. **Me llamo Alexander.**
[meh ya-mo Alexander]

You put on the shoes. **Te pones los zapatos.**
[teh pon-es los za-pat-os]

They put on the bandage. **Se pone el vendaje.**
[se po-neh el ben-da-heh]

We feel sick. **Nos sentimos enfermos.** [nos sen-tee-mos en-fer-mos]

You all remember the question. **Os acordáis la pregunta.** [os ak-or-dice la preh-goon-tah]

They go to the hospital. **Se van al hospital.** [se ban al os-pee-tal]

MORE VERB TENSES

Verb tense is an important part of communication, as it allows you to express when exactly an event occurs. Up to this point, we have conjugated commonly used verbs (regular, irregular, and reflexive) in the present tense. This next section includes verb conjugations for a few more verb tenses in Spanish. Each tense will include the endings for **-ar, -er, and -ir** verbs. While this does not cover all tenses, it covers some that you are most likely to use. At the end of the book is *Part 6: Continuing Education*, where you can find resources for learning more about verb conjugation.

Preterite Tense

The preterite tense in Spanish is a form of the past tense. It is used to describe actions or events that were completed in the past. An important thing to know about the preterite tense is that it is used to describe actions or events with a definite beginning and ending, or in other words, a completed action. For example, "I drove my car yesterday." This implies that the action (of driving a car) was a past event with a definite beginning and ending (yesterday).

-AR Endings

Yo *I*	é	Nosotros (as) _{We}	**amos**
Tú *you*	**aste**	Vosotros (as) _{You all}	**asteis**
Él/ Ella/ Usted _{He/ She/ You formal / It}	ó	Ellos/ Ellas/ Ustedes _{You all/They}	**aron**

-ER Endings

Yo *I*	í	Nosotros (as) _{We}	**imos**
Tú *you*	**iste**	Vosotros (as) _{You all}	**isteis**
Él/ Ella/ Usted _{He/ She/ You formal / It}	**ió**	Ellos/ Ellas/ Ustedes _{You all/They}	**ieron**

-IR Endings

Yo *I*	í	Nosotros (as) _{We}	**imos**
Tú *you*	**iste**	Vosotros (as) _{You all}	**isteis**
Él/ Ella/ Usted _{He/ She/ You formal / It}	**ió**	Ellos/ Ellas/ Ustedes _{You all/They}	**ieron**

Notice that the verb endings for **-er and -ir** preterite verbs are the **same**.

Imperfect Tense

The imperfect tense is similar to the preterite tense, in that it is used to refer to past events; however, it is used in slightly different contexts. The imperfect tense is used to talk about **habitual** past events. For example, "She used to go to the doctor every week when she was a child." The key phrase in this sentence is "used to", as it implies a past habitual event. Another use for the imperfect is to describe what someone was doing when they were interrupted by something else. For example, "I was walking [imperfect] when suddenly, I fell [preterite]."

-AR Endings

Yo *I*	**aba**	Nosotros (as) *We*	**ábamos**
Tú *You*	**abas**	Vosotros (as) *You all*	**abais**
Él/ Ella/ Usted *He/ She/ You formal/ It*	**aba**	Ellos/ Ellas/ Ustedes *You all/They*	**aban**

-ER Endings

Yo /	ía	Nosotros (as)	íamos
Tú *You*	ías	Vosotros (as) *You all*	íais
Él/ Ella/ Usted	ía	Ellos/ Ellas/ Ustedes	ían

-IR Endings

Yo /	ía	Nosotros (as) *We*	íamos
Tú *You*	ías	Vosotros (as) *You all*	íais
Él/ Ella/ Usted *He/ She/ You formal / It*	ía	Ellos/ Ellas/ Ustedes *You all/They*	ían

Future Tense

The simple future tense is used to talk about things that *will* happen. For example, I *will* go to the store. To properly conjugate a verb in the future tense, take the infinitive form of the verb and without taking off the verb endings, add the future tense ending. For example, hablar (to talk) become hablaré (I will talk).

-AR Endings, -ER Endings, -IR Endings

Yo *I*	**é**	Nosotros (as) *We*	**emos**
Tú *You*	**ás**	Vosotros (as) *You all*	**éis**
Él/ Ella/ Usted *He/ She/ You formal/ It*	**á**	Ellos/ Ellas/ Ustedes *You all/They*	**án**

Examples:

I will walk. **Caminaré.** [kam-een-ar-é]

You will eat. **Comerás.** [kom-er-ás]

He will go. **Irá.** [eer-á]

We will sleep. **Dormiremos.** [dor-meer-emos]

You all will hear. **Escucharéis.** [es-ku-char-éis]

They will learn. **Aprenderán.** [ap-ren-der-án]

Informal or Near Future Tense

The informal future tense is used to say that you are "going to do" something. For example, "I am going to go to the hospital." The informal future tense is commonly used in conversational Spanish. To form a sentence in the informal future tense, use the following structure.

Ir (*to go*) + a (*to*) + infinitive verb

IR + A + INFINITIVE

To create a sentence using the informal future tense, conjugate the desired form of the verb "**ir**" (to go), then add the word "**a**" (to) and finally place the infinitive form of the desired verb. Remember that an infinitive verb is the unconjugated form.

Ir *(to go)*

Yo I	**voy**	Nosotros (as) _{We}	**vamos**
Tú _{You}	**vas**	Vosotros (as) _{You all}	**vais**
Él, Ella, Usted _{He/ She/ You formal / It}	**va**	Ellos/ Ellas/ Ustedes _{You all/They}	**van**

Examples:

I am going to go to the hospital. **Voy a ir al hospital.** [boy a eer al os-pit-al]

You are going to call the police. **Vas a llamar a la policía.** [bas a yam-ar a la pol-ee-sía]

She is going to look for help. **Ella va a buscar ayuda.** [eya ba a bus-kar ay-oo-dah]

We are going to run. **Nosotros vamos a correr.** [nos-oh-tros ba-mos a kor-rer]

You all are going to leave. **Vosotros vais a salir.** [vos-oh-tros bais a sal-eer]

They are going to help. **Ustedes van a ayudar.** [oos-ted-es bahn a ay-oo-dar]

NUMBERS

Knowing how to say numbers in Spanish is a simple yet essential part of communication. Numbers that range from zero through twenty-nine require memorization; however, once memorized, numbers above twenty-nine are characterized by a pattern that is easy to follow.

ONES

0	Cero
1	Uno/Un/Una
2	Dos
3	Tres
4	Cuatro
5	Cinco
6	Seis
7	Siete
8	Ocho
9	Nueve

TEENS

10	Diez
11	Once
12	Doce
13	Trece
14	Catorce
15	Quince
16	Dieciséis
17	Diecisiete
18	Dieciocho
19	Diecinueve

TWENTIES

20	Veinte
21	Veintiuno/-un/-una
22	Veintidós
23	Veintitrés
24	Veinticuatro
25	Veinticinco
26	Veintiséis
27	Veintisiete
28	Veintiocho
29	Veintinueve

THIRTIES

30	Treinta
31	Treinta y uno/un/una
32	Treinta y dos
33	Treinta y tres
34	Treinta y cuatro
35	Treinta y cinco
36	Treinta y seis
37	Treinta y siete
38	Treinta y ocho
39	Treinta y nueve

Numbers continue to follow the pattern where the tens digit remains the same and the ones digit changes and is separated by the word "y" which means **and**. For example, fiftyeight is "cincuenta y ocho".

TENS

10	Diez
20	Veinte
30	Treinta
40	Cuarenta
50	Cincuenta
60	Sesenta
70	Setenta
80	Ochenta
90	Noventa

HUNDREDS

100	Cien
200	Doscientos/-as
300	Trescientos/-as
400	Cuatrocientos/-as
500	Quinientos/-as
600	Seiscientos/-as
700	Setecientos/-as
800	Ochocientos/-as
900	Novecientos/-as

THOUSANDS +

1,000	Mil
10,000	Diez mil
100,000	Cien mil
1,000,00	Un millón
10,000,000	Diez millón
100,000,000	Cien millón

Take note that in many countries, including Spanish speaking countries, the comma and period are switched in regard to numbers. 10,000 (ten thousand) is written as 10.000. Likewise, numbers with decimal points also switch. As an example, 3.47 (three point forty seven) is written as 3,47.

Ordinal Numbers

Number	Spelling
1°	Primero (a)
2°	Segundo (a)
3°	Tercero (a)
4°	Cuarto (a)
5°	Quinto (a)
6°	Sexto (a)
7°	Séptimo (a)
8°	Octavo (a)
9°	Noveno (a)
10°	Décimo (a)

Common Questions & Responses

Listed below are a couple of number related questions and responses that are most pertinent to the field of Emergency Medical Services. They are modeled using the formal you, *usted*.

1:

How much do you weigh? **¿Cuánto pesa?** [kuán-toh pe-sa]

I weigh 150 pounds/kilograms. **Yo peso 150 libras/kilogramos.** [yo pe-so see-ehn-toh seen-kwen-tah lee-bras/ keel-o-gram-os]

2:

What time is it? **¿Qué hora es?** [keh o-rah es]
It's 3 o'clock. **Son las tres.** [son las tres]

3:

How many drinks have you had? **¿Cuántas bebidas ha tomado?** [kuán-tas beh-bee-das ah tom-ado]
I've had three drinks. **He tomado tres bebidas.** [eh tom-ado tres beh-bee-das]

4:

How old are you? **¿Cuántos años tiene?** [kuán-tos anyos tee-eh-ne]
I am 25 years old. **Tengo 25 años.** [ten-go bein-tee-seen-koh anyos]

5:

When did this happen? **¿Hace cuánto pasó esto?** [ah-seh kuán-to pa-só es-to]
It happened 40 minutes ago. **Pasó hace 40 minutos.** [pa-só ah-seh kuar-en-tah min-oo-tos]

6:

When did the pain start? **¿Cuándo empezó el dolor?** [kuán-do em-peh-zó el dol-or]
The pain started ten minutes ago. **El dolor empezó hace diez minutos.** [el dol-or em-pe-zó ah-seh dee-ez min-oo-tos]

Conclusion: Spanish Language Basics

The alphabet, basic grammar rules, and simple vocabulary words were the main focus of this section. Whether this was a review or brand new information, you should now have the basic linguistic knowledge that will help you accelerate your learning in the following sections.

Part 2: Greetings & Commonly Used Language

As you begin this next section, it will be important for you to use the information provided in *Part 1: Spanish Language Basics* as a guide and reference point. This section includes some of the most common phrases, including: greetings, asking "how are you?", and other essential words. The latter part of this section includes a few simple practice examples using the vocabulary from this section.

Common Greetings

English	Spanish	Phonetic Pronunciation
Hello	Hola	oh-la
Good morning	Buenos días	bweh-nos dee-as
Good afternoon	Buenas tardes	bweh-nas tar-des
Good evening	Buenas noches	Bweh-nas noch-es
What's your name? informal	¿Cómo te llamas?	kó-mo te yam-as
What's your name? formal	¿Cómo se llama?	kó-mo se yam-ah
It's nice to meet you informal	Mucho gusto	moo-cho goos-toh
It's nice to meet you formal	Encantado (a) de conocerle	en-can-ta-doh deh kono-ser-leh
Likewise	Igualmente	ee-gwal-mehn-teh

Asking, "How are you?"

English	Spanish	Phonetic Pronunciation
How are you? *informal*	¿Cómo estás?	kó-mo es-tás
How are you? *formal*	¿Cómo está usted?	kó-mo es-ta oos-ted
How's it going?	¿Cómo te va?	kó-mo teh ba
How have you been?	¿Cómo te ha ido?	kó-mo teh ah ee-doh
What's up?	¿Qué tal?	keh tal
What's happening	¿Qué pasa?	keh pa-sah
What are you doing?	¿Qué haces?	keh ah-ses

Responses

English	Spanish	Phonetic Pronunciation
Well, thanks.	Bien, gracias.	bee-en gras-ee-as
Very well.	Muy bien.	Muy bee-en
And you?	¿Y tú?	ee too
As always.	Como siempre.	ko-mo see-em-preh
I'm a little tired.	Estoy un poco cansado (a).	ehs-toy un po-ko kahn-sah-doh
I don't feel well.	No me siento bien.	no meh see-en-toh bee-en
I'm sick.	Estoy enfermo (a).	es-toy en-fer-moh
Okay, so-so	Más o menos.	más oh meh-nos
Bad.	Mal.	mal
Well.	Bien.	bee-en
Nothing.	Nada.	na-dah

Saying Goodbye

English	Spanish	Phonetic Pronunciation
Goodbye.	Adiós.	ah-dee-os
Until later.	Hasta luego.	ahs-tah lu-eh-go
See you soon.	Hasta pronto.	ahs-tah pron-toh
Until next time.	Hasta la vista.	ahs-tah la bee-stah
See you.	Nos vemos.	nos beh-mos

Essential Phrases

English	Spanish	Phonetic Pronunciation
Yes	Sí	see
No	No	noh
Thank you.	Gracias.	gra-see-as
You're welcome.	De nada.	deh nada
Please.	Por favor.	por fa-vor
I'm sorry.	Lo siento.	lo see-en-toh
I'm sorry.	Disculpa.	dis-cul-pah
Do you need help?	¿Necesitas ayuda?	nes-eh-sitas ay-oo-dah
I need help.	Necesito ayuda.	nes-eh-sito ay-oo-dah
Help me!	¡Ayúdame!	ayoo-da-meh
Help!	¡Socorro!	sok-oro
Excuse me.	Con permiso.	kon per-me-soh
What a shame.	¡Que lástima!	keh lá-stee-mah

Directional

English	Spanish	Phonetic Pronunciation
Above	Encima de	en-see-mah
Around	Sobre	soh-breh
Behind	Detrás (de)	deh-trás (deh)
Below	Debajo (de)	deh-baho (deh)
Inside (of)	Dentro	den-troh (deh)
Close (to)	Cerca (de)	ser-kah (deh)
In front (of)	Enfrente (de)	en-fren-teh (deh)
Far	Lejos	le-hos
Left	Izquierda	eez-kee-er-dah
Outside (of)	Fuera (de)	foo-er-ah (deh)
On top (of)	En la cima (de)	en la see-mah (deh)
Right	Derecha	der-eh-cha
Straight	Derecho	der-eh-cho

Examples with directional words:

Is the hospital close? **¿Está cerca el hospital?** [es-tá ser-kah el os-pee-tal]

The medicine is to the left. **La medicina está a la izquierda.** [la medi-seen-ah es-tá a la eez-kee-er-dah]

There is a dog outside of the house. **Hay un perro fuera de la casa.** [ay un per-roh foo-er-ah de la ka-sa]

There is a knife behind me. **Hay un cuchillo detrás de mí.** [ay un ku-chee-oh de-trás de me]

Temporal

English	Spanish	Phonetic Pronunciation
Second	El segundo	el seg-oon-doh
Minute	El minuto	el min-oo-toh
Hour	La hora	la or-ah
Today	Hoy	oy
Tomorrow	Mañana	ma-nya-na
Yesterday	Ayer	ay-er
Last night	Anoche	a-no-cheh
Tomorrow night	Mañana por la noche	ma-nya-na por la no-cheh
Week	La semana	la se-man-ah
Last week	La semana pasada	la se-man-ah pas-ah-dah
Next week	La próxima semana	la próx-ee-mah se-man-ah
Next month	El próximo mes	el próx-ee-mo mes
[A month] ago	Hace [un mes]	ah-seh [un mes]

Examples with temporal words:

The pain started ten minutes ago. **El dolor empezó hace diez minutos.** [el dol-or em-peh-zó ah-seh dee-ez min-oo-tos]

I went to the hospital a month ago. **Fui al hospital hace un mes.** [fwi al os-pee-tal ah-seh un mes]

The accident happened five minutes ago. **El accidente pasó hace cinco minutos.** [el ax-ee-den-teh pa-só ah-seh sin-ko min-oo-tos]

My chest pain started yesterday. **Mi dolor de pecho comenzó ayer.** [mee dol-or de peh-cho kom-en-zó ay-er]

I will go to the hospital tomorrow. **Iré al hospital mañana.** [ir-é al os-pee-tal ma-nya-na]

Days of the Week

English	Spanish *(are not capitalized)*	Phonetic Pronunciation
Monday	lunes	loo-nes
Tuesday	martes	mar-tes
Wednesday	miércoles	mee-ér-kol-es
Thursday	jueves	hue-bes
Friday	viernes	bee-er-nes
Saturday	sábado	sá-boh-doh
Sunday	domingo	dom-een-goh

Months

English	Spanish *(are not capitalized)*	Phonetic Pronunciation
January	enero	en-er-oh
February	febrero	feb-rer-oh
March	marzo	mar-zoh
April	abril	ab-reel
May	mayo	mai-yoh
June	junio	hoon-ee-oh
July	julio	hool-ee-oh
August	agosto	ag-os-toh
September	septiembre	sept-ee-em-breh
October	octubre	ok-toob-reh
November	noviembre	nob-ee-em-breh
December	diciembre	dee-see-em-breh

Interaction Examples

Use this section to acquaint yourself with conversation starters and basic communication. There will not be an English translation next to each phrase because the goal at this point is to push you a step further and begin memorization; however, you can reference the tables above to guide you through this section. After each interaction is a brief synopsis that explains why certain words and conjugations were used and how they can be applied in real life situations.

1:

¡Hola Alex! ¿Cómo estás?
Estoy bien, gracias. ¿Cómo estás?
No me siento bien.
Lo siento, Alex. ¿Por qué no te sientes bien?
Estoy enfermo.

> From the beginning of this example, it is clear that the two speakers know each other. The first speaker addresses the second speaker by his name *and* uses the "tú" form of the verb *estar*.

2:

Hola, me llamo Carla. ¿Cómo se llama?
Hola, soy Martin. Encantado de conocerle.
Hola Martin. ¿Cómo está?
¡Estoy bien, gracias! ¿Y usted?
Muy bien, gracias.

> We know that Carla and Martin are strangers when they first meet because they ask for each other's names. They both use the formal form of "you" which is *usted*, as a reminder. Remember that the formal use of "you" is used between acquaintances and professional settings.

3:

Buenos días, Gabriel.
Hola, Marie. ¿Cómo estás?
Mal, no me siento bien.
¡Que lástima! ¿Necesitas ayuda?
No, no gracias.

> From the beginning of this interaction, it is obvious that Gabriel and Marie are friends because they address each other by each other's names. The informal use of you (tú) is used, which indicates friendship. Remember that the

informal use of "you" is used between friends.

4:

Hola, me llamo Emily. ¿Cómo se llama?
Hola Emily, soy Justin.
¿Cómo se siente?
No me siento bien, y necesito ayuda.

In this brief interaction, Emily and Justin are meeting each other for the first time. Since they are strangers meeting for the first time, the verbs are conjugated into the formal "you" (usted) form to indicate formality and give a sense of respect.

Conclusion: Greetings & Commonly Used Language

After completing *Part 2: Greetings & Commonly Used Language* you should now know common greetings and responses, temporal and directional words, days of the week, essential phrases, and more. Having a strong foundation will accelerate your ability to communicate and facilitate your learning in the following sections.

Part 3: Assessment & Intervention

The following section will cover the topic of assessment and intervention along with other pertinent information for the Paramedic, EMT, and Dispatcher. At this point, you should have an adequate base knowledge of Spanish and know how to communicate on a very basic level. This section goes beyond the beginning stages of language learning and will push you a step further. Included in this section are: commonly asked questions, responses, commands and other pertinent information.

In Paramedic and EMT school, we learn certain acronyms for assessing patients and remembering specific information. These acronyms include but are not limited to: BSI, OPQRST, SAMPLE, DCAP BTLS, Alert and Oriented questions, and more. This section will include a translation for each of these acronyms and other related questions and responses. Included in this section will be "textbook" patient assessment questions and responses.

BSI

Body, Substance, Isolation

BODY El cuerpo

SUBSTANCE La sustancia

ISOLATION El aislamiento

Questions:

Are you sick?
> **¿Estás enfermo?** [es-tás en-fer-moh]

Have you been coughing?
> **¿Has tenido tos?** [as ten-ee-doh tos]

Do you have HIV/AIDS/Hepatitis?
> **¿Tienes VIH/SIDA/Hepatitis?** [tee-en-es eh-pah-tee-tees]

Do you have anything that can poke, cut, or shoot me?
> **¿Tienes algo con lo que me pudieras clavar, cortar, o disparar?**
> [tee-en-es al-goh kon lo keh meh pood-ee-er-as kla-var, kor-tar, oh dees-par-ar]

Do you use intravenous drugs?
> **¿Usas drogas intravenosas?** [oo-sas dro-gas een-tra-ben-osas]

Is anyone else in the house/apartment/building right now?

¿Hay alguien más en la casa/apartamento/edificio en este momento? [ay al-gee-en más en la ka-sa/ap-ar-ta-men-toh/ed-ee-fee-see-oh en es-teh mo-men-toh]

Are there any animals here?

¿Hay animales aquí? [ay an-ee-mal-es ah-key]

Common Responses:

Yes, I am sick.

Sí, estoy enfermo (a). [see, es-toy en-ferm-oh(ah)]

No, I am not sick.

No, no estoy enfermo (a). [noh, noh es-toy en-ferm-oh(ah)]

I have Human Immunodeficiency Virus.

Tengo el virus de inmunodeficiencia (VIH). [ten-go el beer-oos de een-moon-oh-deh-fee-see-en-see-ya]

I'm not sure what illness I have.

No estoy seguro cuál es la enfermedad que tengo. [no es-toy seg-oo-roh kwál es la en-ferm-eh-dad keh ten-go]

Yes, I use intravenous drugs.

Sí, uso drogas intravenosas. [see, oo-soh dro-gas een-tra-ben-oh-sas]
No, I do not use intravenous drugs.
No, no uso drogas intravenosas.
[no, no oo-soh dro-gas een-tra-ben-oh-sas]

Yes, there is someone in the house/apartment/building.
Sí, hay alguien más en la casa.
[see, ay al-gee-en más en la ka-sa]
Yes, I have a dog.
Sí, tengo un perro. [see, ten-go un per-roh]
No, I do not have any pets.
No, no tengo ninguna mascota.
[no, no ten-go neen-goon-ah mas-ko-tah]

Statements:
I'm going to put a mask on you.
Te voy a poner un cubre boca. [teh boy a pon-er un koo-breh bo-kah]
Can you cover your cough?
¿Puedes cubrir tu boca al toser?
[pweh-des koo-breer too bo-kah al tos-er]
We are waiting until the police arrive.

Estamos esperando a que llegue la policía. [es-ta-mos es-per-an-doh a keh yeg-eh la pol-ee-see-ah]

Take everything out of your pockets.

Saca todo lo que tengas de tus bolsillos. [sa-kah to-do lo keh ten-gas de toos bol-see-ohs]

Put your dogs/pets in another room.

Pon a tus perros/mascotas en otro cuarto. [pon a toos per-rohs/mas-ko-tahs en oh-tro koo-ar-toh]

OPQRST

Onset, Provocation, Quality, Radiation, Severity, Time

ONSET La aparación

Questions:
Did the pain start suddenly or gradually?
> **¿El dolor comenzó inmediatamente o parcialmente?**
> [el dol-or kom-em-zó in-med-ee-ata-men-teh oh par-see-al-men-teh]

What were you doing when your pain started?
> **¿Qué estabas haciendo cuando el dolor comenzó?** [keh es-ta-bas ah-see-en-doh kwán-do el dol-or kom-em-zó]

Common Responses:
My pain started gradually.
> **El dolor comenzó parcialmente.** [el dol-or kom-en-zó par-see-al-men-teh]

My pain started suddenly.
> **El dolor comenzó inmediatamente.** [el dol-or kom-en-zó in-med-ee-at-ah-men-teh]

I don't know when my pain started.
> **No sé cuando comenzó el dolor.**
> [no seh kwán-do kom-en-zó el dol-or]

PROVOCATION La provocación

Questions:

What makes your pain feel better or worse?
> **¿Qué hace mejorar o empeorar el dolor?** [keh ah-seh me-hor-ar o ehm-peh-or-ar el dol-or]

What provokes the pain?
> **¿Qué provoca el dolor?** [keh pro-bo-ka el dol-or]

Common Responses:

Sitting makes the pain better.
> **Sentarme disminuye el dolor.** [sen-tar-meh dis-men-oo-yeh el dol-or]

Standing makes the pain worse.
> **Pararme empeora el dolor.** [par-ar-meh em-pe-ora el dol-or]

Pressure makes it worse.
> **La presión empeora el dolor.** [la pre-sión em-pe-ora el dol-or]

I feel better if I lay down.
> **Me siento mejor si me acuesto.** [meh see-en-toh me-hor see meh ah-kweh-stoh]

QUALITY La propiedad

Questions:

Is your pain sharp?
> **¿El dolor se siente como una punzada?** [el dol-or seh see-en-teh kó-mo una pun-za-dah]

Is your pain dull?
> **¿El dolor es leve?** [el dol-or es le-beh]

Can you describe your pain?
> **¿Puedes describir el dolor?** [pwe-des des-kreeb-eer el dol-or]

What does your pain feel like?
> **¿Cómo se siente el dolor?** [kó-mo se see-en-teh el dol-or]

Common Responses:

The pain is sharp.
> **El dolor se siente como una punzada.** [el dol-or se see-en-teh kó-mo una pun-za-dah]

The pain is dull.
> **El dolor es leve.** [el dol-or es le-beh]

The pain feels tight.
> **El dolor es tenso.** [el dol-or es ten-so]

The pain is intense/strong.
> **El dolor es intenso/fuerte.** [el dol-or es ten-so/fuer-teh]

I can't describe my pain.

No puedo describir mi dolor. [no pwe-doh des-kreeb-eer mee do-lor]

RADIATION La radiación

Questions:

Does your pain radiate?
¿El dolor se está extendiendo? [el dol-or se es-tá ex-ten-dee-en-doh]

Can you show me where it hurts the most?
¿Me puedes mostrar en dónde está el dolor? [meh pue-des mos-trar en dón-de es-tá el dol-or]

Where else do you have pain?
¿Dónde más sientes dolor? [dón-de más see-en-tes dol-or]

Common Responses:

The pain radiates to my arm.
El dolor se está extendiendo hacia mi brazo. [el dol-or se es-tá ex-ten-dee-en-doh ah-see-ya mee bra-zo]

I have pain around my whole body.
Tengo dolor en todo el cuerpo. [ten-go dol-or en to-do el ku-er-poh]

It hurts most here.
Aquí es donde más me duele. [ah-kee es dón-de más meh dwe-le]

I only have pain here.
>　**Sólo tengo dolor aquí.** [só-lo ten-go dol-or ah-key]

SEVERITY La gravedad

Questions:

Can you rate your pain on a scale from one to ten? Ten is the most pain you have ever experienced.
>　**¿Me puedes decir cuánto te duele en una escala del uno al diez? Considerando que diez es el dolor más fuerte que has sentido.** [meh pwe-des de-seer kuán-to te due-le en una es-ka-lah del oo-no a dee-ez. Kon-sid-er-ando keh dee-ez es el dol-or mas fuer-teh keh as sen-tee-do]

Common Responses:

I have a lot of pain.
>　**Tengo mucho dolor.** [ten-go moo-cho do-lor]

I have a little bit of pain.
>　**Tengo dolor ligero.** [ten-go dol-or lee-her-oh]

TIME El tiempo

Questions:

How long ago did your pain start?
> **¿Hace cuánto empezó el dolor?**
> [ah-seh kwán-to em-peh-zó el dol-or]

When did your pain start?
> **¿Cuándo empezó el dolor?** [kwán-do em-peh-zó el dol-or]

Common Responses:

I was sleeping when my pain started.
> **Estaba durmiendo cuando me empezó a doler.** [es-taba dur-meh-en-doh kwán-do meh em-peh-zó el dol-or]

The pain started three days ago.
> **El dolor comenzó hace tres días.**
> [el dol-or kom-en-zó ah-sey tres dee-as]

The pain started ten minutes ago.
> **El dolor comenzó hace diez minutos.** [el dol-or kom-en-zó ah-sey dee-ez min-oo-tos]

SAMPLE

Signs/Symptoms, Allergies, Medication, Past Pertinent History, Last Intake, Events Leading Up

SIGNS & SYMPTOMS Los indicios y síntomas

Questions:

What symptoms are you experiencing?
> **¿Qué síntomas estás experimentando?** [keh seen-toh-mas es-tás ex-per-ee-men-tan-doh]

What are you feeling right now?
> **¿Qué estás sintiendo en este momento?** [keh es-tás sin-tee-en-doh en es-te mo-men-toh]

Why did you call for an ambulance?
> **¿Por qué llamaste a una ambulancia?** [por keh yam-as-teh a oo-na ambu-lan-sia]

What can I do to make you feel better?
> **¿Qué puedo hacer para hacerte sentir mejor?** [keh pwe-doh ah-ser pa-ra ah-ser-teh sen-teer me-hor]

Common responses:

I feel sick.
> **Me siento enfermo.** [meh see-en-toh en-fer-moh]

I want to kill myself.
> **Quiero matarme.** [key-er-oh mat-ar-meh]

My chest feels tight.
> **Mi pecho siente una presión.** [mee pe-cho see-en-teh una pren-sión]

My head really hurts.
> **Me duele mucho la cabeza.** [meh dwe-le moo-cho la ka-beh-za]

I can't feel my legs.
> **No puedo sentir mis piernas.** [no pwe-do sen-teer mees pee-er-nas]

It's hard to breath.
> **Es difícil respirar.** [es dee-fee-seel res-peer-ar]

I passed out.
> **Me desmayé.** [meh des-mai-éh]

I'm having an allergic reaction.
> **Estoy teniendo una reacción alérgica.** [es-toy ten-ee-en-doh una re-ak-see-ón al-er-hee-kah]

ALLERGIES Las alergias

Questions:

Do you have any allergies?
> **¿Tienes alguna alergia?** [tee-en-es al-goon-ah al-er-hee-ah]

Are you allergic to any foods, medications, or insects?
> **¿Eres alérgico(a) a algún alimento, medicina o insectos?** [er-es al-er-hee-koh a al-goon al-ee-men-toh, medi-seen-ah, oh in-sek-tohs]

Do you have any allergies we should know about?
> **¿Tienes alguna alergia que deberíamos saber?** [tee-en-es al-goon-ah al-er-hee-ah keh de-ber-ee-ah-mos sa-ber]

Common Responses:

I am allergic to Aspirin.
> **Soy alérgico(a) a la aspirina.** [soy al-er-hee-ko a la as-peer-ee-na]

I am allergic to peanuts.
> **Soy alérgico(a) al maní.** [soy al-er-hee-ko al mah-nee]

I am not allergic to anything.
> **No soy alérgico(a) a nada.** [no soy al-er-hee-ko a na-da]

I don't know what I am allergic to.
> **No sé a que soy alérgico(a)** [no seh a keh soy al-er-hee-ko]

I'm allergic to some medicine, but I don't know which.

Soy alérgico(a) a una medicina pero no sé cuál. [soy al-er-hee-ko a una medi-seen-ah pe-roh no seh kwál]

MEDICATIONS Las medicaciones

Questions:

Are you prescribed any medications?
¿Tienes recetado algún medicamento? [tee-en-es re-se-tado al-goon medi-ka-mento]

Do you take any medications?
¿Tomas algún medicamento? [to-mas al-goon meh-dee-ka-mento]

Do you take any medications that are not prescribed to you?
¿Tomas algún medicamento sin receta? [to-mas al-goon meh-dee-ka-mento seen re-se-ta]

Common Responses:

I don't know what medications I am on.
No sé qué medicamentos tomo. [no seh keh meh-dee-ka-mento to-mo]

Yes, I take <u>Aspirin</u> every day.
Sí, tomo aspirina todos los días. [see to-mo as-pri-na to-dos los dí-as]

I take medications when I need it.

Tomo medicamentos cuando lo necesito. [to-mo meh-dee-ka-mento kwán-do lo nes-eh-see-to]

PERTINENT MEDICAL HISTORY El historial médico pertinente

Questions:

Do you have any medical history?
¿Tienes historial médico? [tee-en-es is-toh-ree-ah meh-dee-ko]

Do you have any medical conditions?
¿Tienes condiciones médicas específicas? [tee-en-es kon-di-see-ón-es meh-dee-kas es-pes-í-fee-kas]

When was the last time you went to the doctor, and why did you go?
¿Cuándo fue la última vez que fuiste al doctor? ¿Por qué fuiste? [kwán-do fue la úl-tee-mah vez keh fwee-steh al dok-tor]

Common Responses:

I had a heart attack last year.
Tuve un ataque de corazón (infarto) el año pasado. [tu-beh un ata-keh de kor-ah-zón el anyo pas-ado]

I do not have any medical conditions.

No tengo ninguna condición médica. [no ten-go neen-goon-ah kon-dee-see-ón meh-dee-ka]

LAST INTAKE La última ingesta

Questions:

When was the last time you ate something?
> **¿Cuándo fue la última vez que comiste algo?** [kwán-do fwe la úl-tee-mah vez keh kom-ee-steh al-go]

When was the last time you drank something?
> **¿Cuándo fue la última vez que bebiste algo?** [kwán-do fwe la úl-tee-mah vez keh beb-ee-steh al-go]

Have you consumed any alcohol?
> **¿Has consumido alcohol?** [as kon-soom-ee-doh al-kol]

Have you taken any drugs?
> **¿Has consumido drogas?** [as kon-soom-ee-doh dro-gas]

Common Responses:

I ate breakfast this morning.
> **Desayuné esta mañana.** [des-ai-oon-é es-ta ma-nya-na]

I drank water last night.
> **Anoche bebí agua.** [a-no-cheh be-bee ag-wa]

I drank two beers.
> **Bebí dos cervezas.** [be-bee dos ser-beh-sas]

No, I have not taken any drugs.
> **No, no he consumido drogas.** [no, no eh kon-soom-ee-doh dro-gas]

EVENTS Los acontecimientos

Questions:

What were you doing before the accident?
> **¿Qué estabas haciendo antes del accidente?** [keh es-ta-bas ah-see-en-doh an-tes del ax-ee-den-teh]

What were you doing when your pain started?
> **¿Qué estabas haciendo cuando comenzó el dolor?** [keh es-ta-bas ah-see-en-doh kwán-do kom-em-zó el dol-or]

What activities have you done today?
> **¿Qué actividades has hecho el día de hoy?** [keh ak-tib-ee-dad-es as eh-cho el dí-a de oy]

Common Responses:

I was sleeping when my pain started.
> **Estaba durmiendo cuando el dolor comenzó.** [es-ta-ba dur-me-en-do kwán-do el dol-or kom-en-zó]

I was outside when I started to feel sick.

Estaba afuera cuando comencé a sentirme enfermo. [es-taba ah-fwera kwán-do kom-en-sé a sen-teer en-fer-moh]

I have been in my house all day today.
He estado todo el día en mi casa.
[eh es-ta-doh to-do el dee-ah en mee ka-sa]

I was riding my bike before the accident.
Estaba montando mi bicicleta antes del accidente. [es-taba mon-tan-do mee bee-see-kle-ta an-tes del ax-ee-den-teh]

I was at a bar before the accident.
Estaba en un bar antes del accidente. [es-taba en un bar an-tes del ax-ee-den-teh]

DCAP BTLS

This part will include the acronym DCAP BTLS along with statements patients might say about their injuries in relation to each word. Note that there is a world of possibility when it comes to how a patient acquired an injury. The responses listed in this section are very basic and common.

Deformity and Dislocation La deformidad y dislocación

I tripped and fell.
> **Me tropecé y me caí.** [meh tro-pe-sé ee meh ka-ee]

I fell off a ladder.
> **Me caí de la escalera.** [meh ka-ee de la es-ka-ler-a]

I was riding my bike when I fell.
> **Estaba montando mi bicicleta cuando me caí.** [es-taba mon-tan-do mi bee-see-kle-ta kwán-do meh ka-í]

Contusion La contusión

I was in a car accident.
> **Estuve en un accidente automovilístico.** [es-tu-beh en un ax-ee-den-teh ow-toh-mo-bil-ee-stee-koh]

Someone hit me.
> **Alguien me golpeó.** [al-gee-en meh gol-peh-ó]

I fell off my bike.

Me caí de mi bicicleta. [meh ka-ee de mee bee-see-kle-ta]

Abrasion La abrasión

I fell off a motorcycle.
Me caí de una motocicleta. [meh ka-ee de una moto-see-kleh-ta]
I slipped and fell.
Me resbalé y me caí. [meh res-bal-é ee meh ka-ee]

Burn La quemadura

I was doing electric work and some wires burned me.
Estaba haciendo trabajo eléctrico y me quemé con los cables. [es-taba ah-see-en-doh tra-ba-ho el-ék-tree-ko ee meh keh-mé kon los kab-les]
Hot water spilled on me.
Me cayó agua caliente. [meh kay-ó ag-wa kal-ee-en-teh]
I got a sunburn.
El sol me causó una quemadura.
[el sol meh kau-só una keh-ma-du-ra]

Tenderness La ternura

My leg is tender because I fell.

Mi pierna está sensible porque me caí. [mee pee-er-na es-tá sen-see-bleh por-keh meh ka-ee]

I hurt my arm in a car accident.
Lastimé mi brazo en un accidente automovilístico. [las-tee-méh mee bra-zo en un ax-ee-den-teh auto-mo-bil-ee-stee-koh]

My back hurts.
Me duele mi espalda. [meh dwe-le me es-pal-da]

Laceration La laceración

Someone cut me with a knife.
Alguien me cortó con un cuchillo. [al-gee-en meh kor-tó kon un koo-chee-oh]

I cut my foot.
Me corté el pie. [meh kor-téh el pee-eh]

I cut my stomach in a car accident.
Me corté mi estómago en un accidente automovilístico. [meh kor-tée mee es-toh-ma-go en un ax-ee-den-teh auto-mo-bil-ee-stee-koh]

Swelling La hinchazón

I was stung by a bee.
Una abeja me picó. [una ah-beh-ha meh pee-kó]

I am allergic to nuts.

Soy alérgico al maní. [soy al-er-hee-ka al ma-ní]

I have congestive heart failure.
Tengo insuficiencia cardíaca congestiva. [ten-go in-soo-fee-see-en-see-ah kar-dí-aka kon-hes-tee-ba]

Alert and Oriented Assessment
Evaluación alerta y orientada

PERSON La persona
Questions:
What is your name?
> **¿Cómo te llamas?** [kó-mo te yam-as]

Common Responses:
My name is <u>Amanda</u>.
> **Mi nombre es Amanda.** [mee nom-breh es Amanda]

I don't know.
> **No sé.** [no séh]

PLACE El sitio
Questions:
Do you know where you are right now?
> **¿Sabes dónde te encuentras en este momento?** [sab-es dón-de te en-kwen-tras en es-te mo-men-toh]

Where are we right now?
> **¿Dónde estamos en este momento?** [dón-de es-ta-mos en es-te mo-men-toh]

Common Responses:

We are at my house.
> **Estamos en mi casa.** [es-ta-mos en mee ka-sa]

We are at the store/bar/restaurant/park/club/concert.
> **Estamos en la tienda/bar/restaurante/parque/club/concierto.** [es-ta-mos en la tee-en-da/bar/rest-ar-ran-teh/par-keh/club/kon-see-er-toh]

I don't know where I am.
> **No sé dónde estoy.** [no séh dón-de es-toy]

TIME El tiempo

Questions:

What is today's date?
> **¿Qué día es hoy?** [keh dee-a es oy]

Do you know what today is?
> **¿Sabes qué día es hoy?** [sab-es keh dee-a es oy]

Common Responses:

Today is Monday, June 8, 2020.
> **Hoy es lunes 8 de junio de 2020.** [oy es loo-nes oh-cho de oon-ee-oh de dos meel bein-teh]

Today is January 25, 2021.

Hoy es 25 de enero de 2021. [oy es benti sin-ko de en-er-oh de dos meel bentee uno]

I don't know what day it is.
No sé qué día es hoy. [no séh keh dee-a es oy]

EVENT El acontecimiento

Questions:

Where are you right now?
¿Dónde estás ahora? [dón-de es-tás ah-ora]

Do you know where you are?
¿Sabes dónde estás? [sab-es dón-de es-tás]

What city are we in right now?
¿En qué ciudad estamos en este momento? [en keh see-oo-dad es-tamos en es-te mo-men-toh]

What state are we in right now?
¿En qué estado estamos en este momento? [en keh es-ta-doh es-tamos en es-te mo-men-toh]

Common Responses:

I am at home/work/school.
Estoy en casa/trabajo/escuela. [es-toy en ka-sa/tra-ba-ho/es-kwe-la]

I am at the bar/club/restaurant/park/concert.

Estoy en el bar/club/restaurante/parque/concierto. [es-toy en el bar/klub/rest-ar-ran-teh/par-keh/kon-see-er-toh]

I am in Denver, Colorado.
Estoy en Denver, Colorado. [es-toy en Denver, Colorado]

I don't know where I am.
No sé en dónde estoy. [no seh en dón-de es-toy]

OTHER

While there is a wide range of questions, responses, and commands that are used within the field of emergency medical services, this book only encompasses some of the most commonly used language. Here are a few more common questions, responses and comments that are helpful for the Paramedic, EMT, and Dispatcher.

Questions:

How are you feeling?
> **¿Cómo te sientes?** [kó-mo te see-en-tes]

When was the accident?
> **¿Cuándo fue el accidente?** [kwán-do fwe el ax-ee-den-teh]

Is anyone else hurt/injured?
> **¿Hay alguien más herido?** [ay al-gee-en más er-ee-doh]

Is anyone else sick?
> **¿Hay alguien más enfermo?** [ay al-gee-en más en-fer-moh]

Would you like to go to the hospital?
> **¿Te gustaría ir al hospital?** [te goos-ta-ree-ah eer al os-pee-tal]

Can you walk?
> **¿Puedes caminar?** [pwe-des kam-een-ar]

Do you need assistance walking?
¿Necesitas asistencia para caminar? [nes-eh-sitas ah-sees-ten-see-ya para kam-een-ar]

Common responses:

I feel confused/sick.
Me siento confundido/enfermo.
[meh see-en-toh kon-foon-dee-doh/en-fehr-moh]

The accident happened a few minutes ago.
El accidente pasó hace algunos minutos. [el ax-ee-den-teh pa-só ah-seh al-goo-nos min-oo-tos]

I am the only one that is sick.
Soy el único que está enfermo.
[soy el oo-nee-koh keh es-tá en-fer-moh]

I am the only one that is injured.
Soy el único que está herido. [soy el oo-nee-koh keh es-tá er-ee-doh]

Yes, there are other people in the accident.
Sí, hay más gente en el accidente.
[see, ay más hen-teh en el ax-ee-den-teh]

Yes, I need help walking.
Sí, necesito ayuda para caminar.
[see, nes-eh-see-toh ay-oo-dah para kam-een-ar]

No, I do not need help walking.
No, no necesito ayuda para caminar. [no, no nes-eh-see-toh ay-oo-dah para kam-een-ar]

Yes, I want to go to the hospital.
> **Sí, quiero ir al hospital.** [see, key-er-oh eer a os-pee-tal]

No, I do not want to go to the hospital.
> **No, no quiero ir al hospital.** [no, no key-er-oh eer al os-pee-tal]

Commands:

You have to go to the hospital.
> **Tienes que ir al hospital.** [tee-en-es keh eer al os-pee-tal]

You have the right to refuse to go to the hospital.
> **Tienes el derecho de negarte a ir al hospital.** [tee-en-es el der-eh-cho de neh-gar-teh ah eer al os-pee-tal]

You cannot refuse to go to the hospital.
> **No puedes negarte a ir al hospital.** [no pwe-des neh-gar-teh a eer al os-pee-tal]

Let's go to the ambulance.
> **Vamos a la ambulancia.** [ba-mos a la ambu-lan-see-ah]

Let's get you checked out in the ambulance.
> **Vamos a checarte en la ambulancia.** [ba-mos a che-kar-te en la ambu-lan-see-ah]

I highly recommend that you go to the hospital.

Te recomiendo mucho que vayas al hospital. [te re-ko-mee-en-doh moo-cho keh bay-as al os-pee-tal]

I don't believe that you need to go to the hospital.

No creo que necesites ir al hospital. [no kre-oh keh nes-eh-see-tes eer al os-pee-tal]

We cannot accept additional people in the ambulance.

No podemos aceptar a más personas en la ambulancia. [no po-de-mos ax-ep-tar a más per-son-as en la ambu-lan-see-ya]

Your family/friends/husband/wife/parents/siblings can meet you at the hospital.

Su familia/amigos/esposo/esposa/padres/hermanos pueden verse en el hospital. [su fam-ee-lya/es-po-so/es-po-sa/pad-res/ehr-man-nos pwe-den ber-se en el os-pee-tal]

Conclusion: Assessment & Intervention

Part 3: Assessment & Intervention included some of the most commonly used questions, responses, and commands. The purpose of this section is to get you— the first responder— accustomed to assessing patients in Spanish with language that is most commonly used. For best results, focus on proper pronunciation by utilizing the phonetic pronunciation section.

Part 4: Vocabulary

By this point you should have a basic understanding of the Spanish language. This next section includes a list of vocabulary words that are commonly used within the field of Emergency Medical Services. You should now know how to create statements, questions, and have basic comprehension skills. Now it's time to develop your Spanish lexicon. Below are lists of words that are commonly used in Emergency Medical Services. Get creative and apply what you've learned from the previous sections to expand your knowledge!

A few things should be noted about the "Phonetic Pronunciation" section. Some letters have accents on them. When pronouncing these letters, it's important to know that the accents add emphasis or a rise in intonation. This helps to retain word meaning. You will notice that some phonetic pronunciations are identical to the actual spelling; this is because it is pronounced exactly as it looks. On the other hand, some phonetic pronunciations seem exaggerated. The purpose of that is to emphasize each individual sound to ensure proper pronunciation.

For organizational purposes and ease of reference, the vocabulary section is organized into eight topics with subsections organized by the most common parts of speech— nouns, verbs, and adjectives. The vocabulary in this section includes the most common words for each topic, but is by no means an exhaustive list. You will find that many of the words overlap into more than one topic. The purpose of keeping the vocabulary list short is to provide you with the most pertinent information without being overwhelming. A shorter list is easier to reference in a hurry if need be.

4.1 Airway, Respiration, & Ventilation

NOUNS

English	Spanish	Phonetic Pronunciation
Air	El aire	el ay-reh
Airway	La vía respiratoria	la bee-ah res-pir-a-tor-ee-ah
Alveoli	El alvéolo	el al-bé-olo
Asthma	El asma	el as-mah
Bag Valve Mask	La máscara de vávula de bolsa de ventilación	la más-car-ah de báb-ula de bol-sah de ben-til-ah-see-ón
Breath	La respiración	la res-pir-ah-see-ón
Bronchi	El bronquio	el bron-key-oh
Bronchioles	El bronquiolo	el bron-key-ol-ee-o
Capillary	El capilar	el kap-ee-lar
Carbon Dioxide	El dióxido de carbono	el di-óxi-do de kar-bo-noh
Carbon Monoxide	El monóxido de carbono	el mon-óxi-doh de kar-bono

Cellular Respiration	La respiración celular	la res-peer-ah-see-ón sel-oo-lar
Chronic Obstructive Pulmonary Disease	La enfermedad pulmonar obstructiva crónica	la en-fer-meh-dad pul-mon-ar ob-stru-ctiva kró-nee-kah
Continuous Positive Airway Pressure	La presión positiva continua en la vía aérea	la pre-sión po-see-tee-ba con-tin-ua en la bía aé-rea
Cricoid Cartilage	El cartílago cricoides	el kart-í-lago kri-koid-es
Diaphragm	El diafragma	el dia-frag-mah
Depth	La profundidad	la pro-foon-dee-dad
Edema	El edema	el ed-eh-mah
Emphysema	El enfisema	el en-fee-seh-mah
Endotracheal Tube	El tubo endotraqueal	el too-boh endo-trak-eh-al
Epiglottis	La epiglotis	la epi-glot-ees
Epiglottitis	La epiglotitis	la epi-glot-eet-ees

Hemothorax	El hemotórax	el he-mo-tó-rax
Gas Exchange	El intercambio de gas	el inter-kam-bio de gas
Hyperoxia	La hiperoxia	la eeper-ox-ee-ah
Hypoxia	La hipoxia	la eepoh-oh-eh-mee-ah
Hypoxemia	La hipoxemia	la eep-ox-eh-mee-ah
Liter	El litro	el lee-tro
Lungs	Los pulmones	los pool-mon-es
Membrane	La membrana	la mem-bra-nah
Mouth	La boca	la bo-kah
Nasal Cannula	La cánula nasal	la kán-oo-la nas-al
Nebulizer	El nebulizador	el nebu-leez-ah-dor
Needle	La aguja	la agu-ha
Needle Decompression	La compresión de la aguja	la kom-preh-see-ón de la agu-ha
Parietal Pleura	La pleura parietal	la ple-urah par-ee-et-al

Pleural Fluid	El líquido pleural	el lí-key-doh ple-oo-ral
Pleural Space	El espacio pleural	el espa-see-oh ple-oo-ral
Pneumothorax	El neumotórax	el numo-toh-rax
Rate	La tasa	la ta-sah
Respiratory Arrest	La parada respiratoria	la par-a-dah res-pir-a-tor-ee-ah
Respiratory Distress	La dificultad respiratoria	la difi-kul-tad res-pir-a-tor-ee-ah
Respiration	La respiración	la res-pir-as-ee-ón
Respiratory Failure	La falla respiratoria	la faya res-pir-a-tor-ia
Snoring	El ronquido	el ron-key-doh
Stethoscope	El estetoscopio	el es-tet-o-scop-ee-oh
Stridor	El estridor	el es-tree-dor
Suction	La succión	la suk-see-on
Tachypnea	La taquipnea	la tak-eep-nea
Throat	La garganta	la gar-gan-tah

Thoracic Cavity	La cavidad torácica	la kab-ee-dad tor-á-sik-a
Thorax	El tórax	el tó-rax
Tongue	La lengua	la len-gua
Trachea	La tráquea	la trak-eh-ah
Oral Cavity	La cavidad oral	la kab-ee-dad or-al
Oropharynx	La orofaringe	la oro-far-ing-heh
Oxygen	El oxígeno	el oxí-hen-oh
Pharynx	La faringe	la far-ing-heh
Ventilator	El ventilador	el ben-til-ah-dor
Visceral Pleura	La pleura visceral	la ple-ur-ah vee-ser-al
Wheezing	La sibilancia	la see-bee-lan-see-ah

VERBS

English	Spanish	Phonetic Pronunciation
Auscultate	Ascultar	as-kul-tar
Breathe	Respirar	res-peer-ar
Close	Cerrar	ser-ar
Cough	Toser	tos-er
Cut	Cortar	kor-tar
Exhale	Exhalar	ex-al-ar
Inhale	Inhalar	in-al-ar
Insert	Insertar	in-ser-tar
Intubate	Intubar	in-too-bar
Listen	Escuchar	es-koo-char
Suction	Succionar	sook-see-on-ar
Open	Abrir	ab-reer
Oxygenate	Oxigenar	oxee-hen-ar
Ventilate	Ventilar	ven-teel-ar

ADJECTIVES

English	Spanish	Phonetic Pronunciation
Absent	Ausente	oq-sen-teh
Blocked	Bloqueado (a)	bloh-keh-ado
Bilateral	Bilateral	bee-lat-er-al
Chest Rise	Elevación torácica	ele-ba-see-ón tor-á-see-kah
Clear	Claro (a)	klar-oh
Closed	Cerrado (a)	ser-ah-doh
Constricted	Restringido (a)	res-treen-hee-doh
Cyanotic	Cianótico (a)	see-an-ó-tee-koh
Deflated	Desinflado (a)	des-een-fla-doh
Even	Equitativo (a)	eh-kee-tat-ee-bo
Fast	Rápido (a)	ráp-ee-doh
Flat	Plano (a)	plah-no
Heavy	Pesado (a)	peh-sah-doh
Intubated	Intubado	in-too-bah-doh
Labored	Fatigoso (a)	fa-tee-go-so

Missing	Ausente	ow-sen-teh
Open	Abierto (a)	ab-ee-er-toh
Tight	Apretado (a)	ah-preh-ta-doh
Uneven	Desigual	des-ee-gwal

4.2 Cardiology

NOUNS

English	Spanish	Phonetic Pronunciation
Anticoagulant	El anticoagulante	el ahn-tee-ko-agu-lan-teh
Aortic Dissection	La disección aórtica	la dee-sec-see-ón ah-ór-tee-kah
Aortic Aneurysm	El aneurisma de aorta	el ah-neh-ur-ees-mah de ah-or-tah
Artery	La arteria	la ar-ter-ee-ah
Automatic External Defibrillator (AED)	El desfibrilador externo automatizado	el des-fee-bree-la-dor ex-ter-noh auto-mah-tee-zah-doh
Blood	La sangre	la san-gre
Blood Pressure	La presión arterial	la pren-see-ón ar-ter-ee-al
Bradycardia	La bradicardia	la bra-dee-kar-dee-ah
Capillary	El capilar	el kap-ee-lar
Cardiac Arrest	El paro cardiaco	el paro kard-ee-ah-ko

Cardiopulmonary Resuscitation (CPR)	La resucitación cardiopulmonar	la res-us-ee-ta-see-ón kar-dee-o-pul-mon-ar
Clot	El coágulo	el ko-á-gu-lo
Congestive Heart Failure	La insuficiencia cardíaca congestiva.	la in-soo-fee-see-en-see-ah kar-dee-ah-kah kon-hes-tee-bah
Diastole	La diástole	la dee-á-sto-le
Dysrhythmia	La disritmia	la dees-reet-mee-ah
Electrocardiogram (EKG)	El electrocardiograma	el eh-lek-tro-kard-ee-oh-grama
Electrodes	El electrodo	el elek-tro-doh
Embolism	La embolia	la embo-lee-ah
Fatigue	La fatiga	la fat-ee-gah
Headache	El dolor de cabeza	el dol-or de ka-beh-zah
Heart	El corazón	el kor-ah-zon
Hyperglycemia	La hiperglucemia	la eeper-glu-seh-mee-ah

Hypertension	La hipertensión	la eeper-ten-see-ón
Hypoglycemia	La hipoglucemia	la eeper-glu-seh-mee-ah
Hypotension	La hipotensión	la eepo-ten-see-ón
Jugular Vein Distention	La distensión de la vena yugular	la dis-ten-sión de la be-na yug-yu-lar
Myocardial Infarction	El infarto de miocardio	el in-fart-oh de mee-o-kard-ee-o
Pressure	La presión	la pren-see-ón
Pulse	El pulso	el pul-soh
Stroke	El accidente cerebrovascular médico	el ax-ee-den-teh ser-ebro-vas-kul-ar méd-ee-koh
Systole	La sístole	la sís-tol-eh
Tachycardia	La taquicardia	la tak-ee-kard-ee-ah
Thrombocyte	El trombocito	el trom-bo-see-tee-o

Vasoconstriction	La vasoconstricción	la baso-kon-strik-see-ón
Vasodilation	La vasodilatación	la baso-di-la-tah-see-ón
Vein	La vena	la be-nah

VERBS

English	Spanish	Phonetic Pronunciation
Bleed	Sangrar	san-grar
Circulate	Circular	seer-ku-lar
Compress	Condensar	kon-den-sar
Defibrillate	Desfibrilar	des-feeb-reel-ar
Depolarize	Despolarizar	des-pol-ar-ee-zar
Feel	Sentir	sen-teer
Palpate	Palpar	pal-par
Put	Poner	pon-er
Repolarize	Repolarizar	re-pol-ee-zar

ADJECTIVES

English	Spanish	Phonetic Pronunciation
Bradycardic	Bradicárdica	brad-ee-kárd-ika
Clammy	Sudado (a)	su-da-doh
Cool	Frío	fr-ío
Decreased	Reducido (a)	re-du-see-doh
Diaphoretic	Diaforético	dia-for-é-tee-ko
Dry	Seco (a)	seh-ko
Elevated	Elevado (a)	eh-leh-vah-doh
Fast	Rápido	rá-pee-doh
Pale	Pálido (a)	pá-lee-doh
Pink	Rosa	ro-sah
Sharp	Afilado (a)	af-ee-lad-oh
Slow	Lento (a)	len-toh
Tight	Ajustado (a)	a-hus-ta-doh
Weak	Débil	dé-beel
Painful	Doloroso (a)	do-lor-oh-so

4.3 Trauma

NOUNS

English	Spanish	Phonetic Pronunciation
Abrasion	La abrasión	la ah-brah-see-ón
Altered Mental Status	El estado mental alterado	el es-ta-doh men-tal al-ter-adoh
Assault	El asalto	el as-al-toh
Bandage	El vendaje	el ben-da-heh
Bicycle	La bicicleta	La bee-see-kle-tah
Burn	La quemadura	la kem-ah-dur-ah
Car	El coche	el ko-cheh
Collision	La colisión	la kol-ee-see-ón
Cramp	El calambre	el ka-lam-breh
Cut	El corte	el kor-teh
Deformity	La deformidad	la de-form-ee-dad
Gauze	La gasa	la gas-ah
Headache	El dolor de cabeza	el dol-or de ka-beh-zah
Impact	El impacto	el im-pact-oh

Knife	El cuchillo	el ku-chee-oh
Laceration	La laceración	la lah-sehr-ah-see-ón
Mechanism of Injury	El mecanismo de la lesión	el mek-an-ees-mo de la leh-see-ón
Motorcycle	La motocicleta	la moto-see-kle-tah
Motor Vehicle Accident	El accidente automovilístico	el ax-ee-den-teh au-toh-mob-ee-lís-tee-koh
Puncture	El pinchazo	el peench-az-ah
Stress	El estrés	el es-trés
Swelling	La hinchazón	la in-chaz-ón
Temperature	La temperatura	la tem-per-ah-tur-ah
Tenderness	La sensibilidad	la sens-ee-beel-ee-dad
Tourniquet	El torniquete	el tor-nee-keh-teh
Triage	El triaje	el tree-ah-heh
Vehicle	El vehículo	el beh-ee-koo-loh
Wound	La herida	la er-ee-dah

VERBS

English	Spanish	Phonetic Pronunciation
Bleed	Sangrar	san-grar
Burn	Quemar	keh-mar
Fall	Caer	kai-er
Hit	Golpear	gol-peh-ar
Kick	Patear	pat-e-ar
Penetrate	Penetrar	pen-eh-trar
Punch	Dar un puñetazo	dar un pun-ye-tah-zoh
Puncture	Pinchar	pin-char
Run	Correr	kor-rer
Shoot	Disparar	dis-par-ar
Stab	Apuñalar	ah-poo-nya-lar
Trip	Tropezar	tro-peh-zar
Walk	Caminar	kam-een-ar
Whack	Golpear	gol-peh-ar

ADJECTIVES

English	Spanish	Phonetic Pronunciation
Aching	Adolorido	ah-do-lor-ee-doh
(A sensation of) Burning	(Una sensación) de ardor	oo-na sens-ah-see-ón de ar-dor
Disoriented	Desorientado (a)	des-or-ee-en-tah-doh (a)
Heavy	Pesado (a)	pe-sah-doh (a)
Hot	Caliente	kal-ee-en-teh
Painful	Doloroso	dol-or-oh-so
Deformed	Deformado (a)	deh-form-ado (a)
Oriented	Orientado (a)	or-ee-en-tah-doh (a)
Sharp	Afilado (a)	af-ee-lah-doh (a)
Tender	Delicado (a)	del-ee-kah-doh
Throbbing	Punzante	poon-zahn-teh
Unconscious	Inconsciente	in-kon-see-en-teh

4.4 Medical

NOUNS

English	Spanish	Phonetic Pronunciation
Acquired Immunodeficiency Syndrome (AIDS)	El síndrome de inmunodeficiencia adquirida (SIDA)	el seen-drom-eh de in-moon-oh-deh-fi-see-en-sya ahd-key-ree-doh
Allergy	La alergia	la al-er-hee-ah
Anaphylaxis	La anafilaxia	la ana-feel-ahx-eea
Bacteria	La bacteria	la bak-ter-eea
Cancer	El cáncer	el kán-ser
Cardiogenic Shock	El shock cardiogénico	el shock kar-dee-oh-hén-ee-ko
Chronic Kidney Disease	La enfermedad renal crónica	la en-fer-me-dad reh-nal krón-ee-kah
Dehydration	La deshidratación	la des-eed-rah-tah-see-ón
Diabetes	La diabetes	la dee-ah-bet-es

Distributive Shock	El shock distributivo	el shock dees-tree-boo-tee-vo
Feces	Las heces	las eh-ses
Hematoma	El hematoma	el ema-toh-ma
Hepatitis	La hepatitis	la eh-pah-tee-tees
Human Immunodeficiency Virus (HIV)	El virus de inmunodeficiencia (VIH)	el beer-oos de in-moon-oh-deh-fee-see-en-sya
Hypovolemic Shock	El shock hipovolémico	el shock ee-poh-bol-émico
Insulin	La insulina	la een-sul-ee-nah
Metabolic Shock	El shock metabólico	el shock meta-ból-ee-ko
Nausea	La náusea	la now-see-ah
Neurogenic Shock	El shock neurogénico	el shock neuro-gén-ee-koh
Obesity	La obesidad	la o-bes-ee-dad
Obstructive Shock	El shock obstructivo	el shock ob-struk-tee-bo
Seizure	El ataque	el ah-tah-keh

Septic Shock	El shock séptico	el shock sép-tee-ko
Tumor	El tumor	el too-mor
Urinary Tract Infection	La infección urinaria	la in-fek-see-ón ur-een-ar-ee-ah
Virus	El virus	el beer-oos

VERBS

English	Spanish	Phonetic Pronunciation
Breathe	Respirar	res-peer-ar
Compensate	Compensar	kom-pen-sar
Constrict	Contraer	kon-trah-er
Cut	Cortar	kor-tar
Dilate	Dilater	dee-la-ter
Dislocate	Dislocar	dis-lok-ar
Decompensate	Descompensar	des-kom-pen-sar
Feel	Sentir	sen-teer
Fracture	Fracturar	frak-toor-ar
Hallucinate	Alucinar	al-oo-seen-ar
Hear	Oir	oi-eer
Ingest	Ingerir	in-her-eer
Perfuse	Perfundir	per-foon-deer
Taste	Probar	pro-bar
Tear	Arrancar	ar-ran-kar
See	Ver	ber
Smell	Oler	ol-er
Strain	Tensar	ten-sar

ADJECTIVES

English	Spanish	Phonetic Pronunciation
Abnormal	Anormal	an-or-mal
Acute	Agudo (a)	ag-oo-doh
Agitated	Agitado (a)	ah-hee-tah-doh
Aggressive	Agresivo (a)	ag-res-ee-boh
Alert	Alerta	al-er-tah
Angry	Enojado (a)	eh-no-ha-doh
Blind	Ciego (a)	see-eh-go
Chronic	Crónico (a)	krón-ee-kah
Confused	Confundido (a)	kon-foon-dee-doh
Deaf	Sordo (a)	sor-doh
Diaphoretic	Diaforético	dee-ah-for-éh-teek-oh
Happy	Feliz	feh-leez
Irreversible	Irreversible	ir-reh-ber-sib-leh
Lethargic	Aletargado (a)	aleh-tar-gah-doh
Nauseous	Con náuseas	kon now-seh-as
Nervous	Nervioso (a)	ner-bee-oh-so
Normal	Normal	nor-mal

Poor	Pobre	pob-reh
Sad	Triste	tree-steh
Septic	Séptico	sép-teek-oh

4.5 Pediatrics

NOUNS

English	Spanish	Phonetic Pronunciation
Adolescent	El/La adolescente	el ad-ol-es-sen-teh
Appendicitis	La apendicitis	la apen-dee-see-tees
Breath holding	Asimiento de la respiración	as-ee-mee-ehn-toh de la res-peer-ah-see-ón
Bronchitis	La bronquitis	la bron-kee-tees
Conjunctivitis (Pink Eye)	La conjuntivitis	la kon-hoon-tee-vee-tees
Colic	El cólico	el kól-ee-ko
Constipation	La constipación	la kon-steep-ah-see-ón
Croup	El crup	el kroop
Developmental Delay	El retraso en el desarrollo	el re-tras-oh en el des-a-roy-o
Diarrhea	La diarrea	la dee-ah-re-ah
Ear Infection	La infección de oído	la in-fek-see-ón de oh-ee-doh
Fever	La fibre	la feeb-reh

Gastroenteritis	La gastroenteritis	la gas-troh-en-ter-ee-tees
Hand-Foot-Mouth Disease	La enfermedad de manos, pies y boca	la en-fer-meh-dad de man-os, pee-ehs, ee bo-kah
Infant	El/La bebé	el beh-béh
Infection	La infección	la in-fek-see-ón
Influenza	La gripe	la gree-peh
Lice	El piojo	el pee-o-ho
Norovirus	El norovirus	el noro-beer-oos
Pertussis (Whooping Cough)	La tos ferina	la tohs fer-ee-nah
Rash	El sarpullido	el sar-pu-yee-doh
Respiratory Syncytial Virus (RSV)	El Virus sincicial respiratorio (VRS)	el beer-oos seen-see-see-al res-peer-a-tor-ee-oh
Shaken Baby Syndrome	El síndrome del niño sacudido	el sín-drom-eh del nee-nyo sa-koo-dee-doh

Side	El lado	el la-doh
Strep	El estreptococo	el es-trep-toh-ko-ko
Sudden Infant Death Syndrome (SIDS)	El síndrome de muerte súbita infantil	el seen-drom de mu-er-teh súb-ee-ta een-fan-teel
Toddler	El niño/la niña	el nee-nyo / la nee-nya

VERBS

English	Spanish	Phonetic Pronunciation
Close	Cerrar	ser-ar
Crawl	Gatear	gat-eh-ar
Cry	Llorar	yor-ar
Defecate	Defecar	deh-feh-kar
Hold	Agarrar	ag-ar-rar
Lift	Levantar	leh-ban-tar
Open	Abrir	ab-reer
Pick Up	Recoger	reh-ko-her
Run	Correr	kor-rer
Set down	Dejar	de-har
Turn	Girar	heer-ar
Urinate	Orinar	or-een-ar
Vomit	Vomitar	bom-ee-tar
Walk	Caminar	kam-een-ar

ADJECTIVES

English	Spanish	Phonetic Pronunciation
Cold	Frío (a)	free-oh
Hot	Caliente	kal-ee-en-teh
Loud	Ruidoso (a)	roo-ee-doh-so
New born	Recién nacido	re-see-én na-see-doh
Persistent	Persistente	per-sis-ten-teh
Warm	Cálido	kál-ee-doh
Quiet	Silencioso (a)	see-len-see-oh-so

4.6 Obstetrics/Gynecology

NOUNS

English	Spanish	Phonetic Pronunciation
Abortion	El aborto	el a-bor-toh
Amniotic fluid	El líquido amniótico	el lee-key-doh am-nee-ó-tee-koh
Breech birth	El parto de nalgas	el par-toh de nal-gas
Cesarean	La cesárea	la ses-ár-eh-ah
Contraction	La contracción	la kon-trak-see-ón
Due date	La fecha de parto	la feh-cha de par-toh
Eclampsia	La eclampsia	la ehk-lamp-see-ah
Embryo	El embrión	el em-bree-ón
Fetus	El feto	el feh-toh
Gestational Diabetes	La diabetes gestacional	la dee-ah-bet-ehs hes-ta-see-ón-al
Labor	El parto	el par-toh
Ovary	El ovario	el o-bar-ee-oh

Placenta	La placenta	la pla-sen-tah
Postpartum Depression	La depresión posparto	la dep-re-see-ón pos-par-toh
Pre-eclampsia	La preeclampsia	la pre-ek-lamp-see-ah
Pregnancy	La gestación	la hes-ta-see-ón
Spontaneous Abortion	El aborto espontáneo	el a-bor-to es-pon-tá-neh-oh
Term	El término	el tér-meen-oh
Trimester	El trimestre	el tree-mes-trey
Umbilical cord	El cordón umbilical	el kor-dón um-beel-eek-al
Uterus	El útero	el oo-ter-oh
Vagina	La vagina	la ba-heen-ah
Womb	La matriz	la mat-reez

VERBS

English	Spanish	Phonetic Pronunciation
Arrive	Llegar	yeg-ar
Contract	Contratarse	kon-trat-ar-seh
Cut	Cortar	kor-tar
Deliver	Atender (el parto)	ah-ten-der (el par-toh)
Induce	Inducir	in-doo-seer
Miscarry	Abortar	ab-or-tar

ADJECTIVES

English	Spanish	Phonetic Pronunciation
Ectopic	Ectópico	ek-tóp-ee-koh
Fetal	Fetal	feh-tal
Hemorrhage	La hemorragia	la eh-moh-rra-hya
Maternity	La maternidad	la mat-er-nee-dad
Overdue	Atrasado (a)	ah-tras-ah-doh
Premature	Prematuro (a)	pre-ma-too-roh
Prenatal	Prenatal	pre-nah-tal
Preterm	Prematuro (a)	pre-ma-too-roh
Unborn	No nacido	noh na-see-doh

4.7 Behavioral, Cognitive, Developmental & Psychiatric

NOUNS

English	Spanish	Phonetic Pronunciation
Addiction	La adicción	la a-dik-see-ón
Alcoholism	El alcoholismo	el al-kol-ees-moh
Alzheimer's Disease	La enfermedad de Alzheimer	la en-fer-mee-dad de Alzheimer
Anorexia Nerviosa	La anorexia nerviosa	la ah-no-rex-ee-ah ner-bee-oh-sah
Anxiety	La ansiedad	la an-see-eh-dad
Aphasia	La afasia	la afa-see-ah
Attention-Deficit Hyperactivity Disorder (ADHD)	El trastorno por déficit de atención e hiperactividad	el tras-tor-no por déh-fee-seet de ah-ten-see-ón ee ee-per-ak-tib-ee-dad
Autism Spectrum Disorder	El trastorno de espectro autista	el tras-tor-no de es-pek-tro ow-tees-ta
Bipolar disorder	El trastorno bipolar	el tras-tor-noh bee-po-lar

Bulimia	La bulimia	la bool-eem-ee-ah
Dementia	La demencia	la deh-men-see-ah
Depression	La depresión	la deh-preh-see-ón
Down Syndrome	El síndrome de Down	el seen-drom-eh de Down
Eating Disorder	El trastorno alimentario	el tras-tor-no ah-lee-men-tar-ee-oh
Homicidal Ideation	El pensamiento homicida	el pen-sa-mee-en-toh oh-me-see-dah
Intoxication	La intoxicación	la een-tox-ee-kah-see-ón
Obsessive Compulsive Disorder	El trastorno obsesivo compulsivo	el tras-tor-no ob-ses-ee-bo com-pool-see-boh
Paranoia	La paranoia	la pah-rah-noy-ah
Personality Disorder	El trastorno de personalidad	el tras-tor-no de per-son-al-ee-dad

Post Traumatic Stress Disorder	El estrés postraumático	el es-trés pos-trau-máh-tee-koh
Schizophrenia	La esquizofrenia	la es-kee-soh-freh-nyah
Suicidal Ideation	El pensamiento suicida	el pen-sa-mee-en-toh swee-see-dah
Withdrawal	El síndrome de abstinencia	el seen-drom-eh de ahbs-tee-nehn-syah

VERBS

English	Spanish	Phonetic Pronunciation
Drink	Beber	beh-ber
Hallucinate	Alucinar	ah-loo-see-nar
Inject	Inyectar	in-yekt-ar
Overdose	Tener una sobredosis	ten-er oo-na sob-re-doh-sees
Sleep	Dormir	dor-meer
Smoke	Fumar	foo-mar

ADJECTIVES

English	Spanish	Phonetic Pronunciation
Absent	Ausente	ow-sen-teh
Abusive	Abusivo (a)	ab-oos-ee-boh
Angry	Enojado (a)	en-oh-ha-doh
Annoyed	Molesto (a)	mol-es-toh
Anxious	Ansioso (a)	ahn-syo-soh
Confused	Confundido (a)	kon-foon-dee-doh
Dependent	Dependiente	de-pen-dee-en-teh
Depressed	Depresivo (a)	deh-pre-see-vo
Nervous	Nervioso (a)	ner-bee-oh-so

4.8 Other Commonly Used Words

NOUNS

English	Spanish	Phonetic Pronunciation
Ambulance	La ambulancia	la ahm-boo-lan-see-ah
Augmentative and Alternative Communication Device	El dispositivo de comunicación aumentativo y alternativo	el dees-pos-ee-tee-vo de kom-oon-ee-kah-see-ón ow-men-tah-tee-bo ee al-ter-na-tee-bo
Bus	El autobus	el ow-toh-boos
Car	El coche	el koh-cheh
Disability	La discapacidad	la dees-kah-pah-see-dad
Disease	La enfermedad	la en-fer-mee-dad
Emergency Department	La sala de emergencia	la sah-lah de em-er-hen-see-ah
Hospital	El hospital	el os-pee-tal
Intravenous Catheter	El catéter intravenoso	el kat-éh-ter intra-ben-oso
Medicine	La medicina	la meh-dee-see-nah

Motorcycle	La motocicleta	la moto-see-kle-tah
Saline	La solución salina	la sol-oo-see-ón sal-ee-nah
Sign Language	La lengua de señas	la len-goo-ah de sen-yas
Stretcher	La camilla	la kam-ee-yah
Vehicle	El vehículo	el beh-hee-koo-loh
Walker	La andadera	la an-dah-der-ah
Wheel chair	La silla de ruedas	la see-ya de roo-eh-das

VERBS

English	Spanish	Phonetic Pronunciation
Abuse	Abusar	ah-boos-ar
Die	Morir	mor-eer
Drink	Beber	beh-ber
Drive	Manejar	man-eh-har
Eat	Comer	kom-er
Pull	Jalar	ha-lar
Push	Empujar	em-poo-har
Rest	Descansar	des-kan-sar
Stop	Parar	par-ar
Talk	Hablar	ah-blar

ADJECTIVES

English	Spanish	Phonetic Pronunciation
Big	Grande	gran-deh
First	Primero (a)	pree-mer-oh
Good	Bueno (a)	boo-eh-noh
Important	Importante	eem-por-tan-teh
Last	Último (a)	ool-tee-moh
Little	Pequeño (a)	peh-ken-yo
Long	Largo	lar-goh
Mute	Mudo	moo-doh
New	Nuevo (a)	noo-eh-boh
Old	Viejo (a)	bee-eh-ho
Short	Corto (a)	kor-toh
Young	Joven	ho-ben

Conclusion: Vocabulary

As you complete *Part 4: Vocabulary*, you should now know some of the most commonly used words related to emergency medical services. As your Spanish lexicon grows, you will be able to communicate more effectively. Having this set of vocabulary will accelerate the communication process which will help you provide better patient care.

Part 5: Dispatch

This section provides some of the most commonly used questions and answers that emergency dispatchers use during a 911 emergency call. The goal of this section is to provide direct Spanish translations that will help dispatchers during a 911 call. Many useful words and phrases can be found in earlier sections, such as: *Part 3: Assessment & Intervention and Part 4: Vocabulary.* While the focus of this book is around Spanish for emergency medical services, this section includes Spanish translations for police and fire emergencies as well. Keep in mind that there is an endless possibility of what people will say during a 911 call, but this section will include some of the most commonly used questions and answers.

WHEN 911 CALLS BEGIN

Questions:
What is the address/location of the emergency?
- **¿Cuál es la dirección/ubicación de la emergencia?** [kwál es la deer-ek-see-ón/oo-bee-ka-see-ón de la eh-mehr-hen-see-ah]

What are the cross streets?
- **¿Entre qué calles?** [en-treh keh ka-yes]

What are nearby landmarks?
- **¿Cuál es el punto de referencia más cercano?** [kwál es el poon-toh deh ref-er-en-see-ah mas ser-kah-noh]

Responses:
What is the phone number you're calling from?
- **¿Cuál es el número de teléfono del que estás marcando?** [kwál es el noo-mer-oh de tel-éh-foh-no del keh es-tás mar-kan-doh]

Do you know what your cell phone number is?
- **¿Sabes cuál es tu número de celular?** [sah-bes kwál es too noo-mer-oh de sel-oo-lar]

Questions:

What is your name?

¿Cómo se llama? (formal) [kó-mo se yah-mah]

What is your name?

¿Cómo te llamas? (informal) [kó-mo te yah-mas]

Responses:

My name is _____.

Me llamo _____. [meh yah-hoh]

I'm _____.

Soy _____. [soy]

Questions:

Can you tell me what exactly happened?

¿Me puedes decir qué pasó exactamente? [meh pweh-des deh-seer keh pa-só ex-ak-ta-men-teh]

Why are you calling 911?

¿Por qué estás llamando a urgencias? [por keh es-tás yah-man-doh a oor-hen-see-ahs]

What is the emergency?

¿Cuál es la emergencia? [kwál es la eh-mer-hen-see-ah]

Responses:

I need to go to the hospital.

Tengo que ir al hospital. [ten-go keh eer al os-pee-tal]

I'm having a medical emergency.
Tengo una emergencia médica. [ten-go una em-er-hen-see-ah méh-dee-ka]

There was an accident.
Hubo un accidente. [oo-boh un ax-ee-den-teh]

I need the police.
Necesito a la policía. [nes-eh-see-toh a la po-lee-see-ah]

Someone has a gun.
Alguien tiene una arma. [al-gee-en tee-eh-heh una ar-mah]

I need firefighters.
Necesito a los bomberos. [nes-eh-see-toh a los bom-ber-os]

There is a fire.
Hay un incendio. [ay un een-sen-dee-oh]

MEDICAL
Questions:
Are you with the patient?
¿Estás con el paciente? [es-tás kon el pah-see-en-teh]

How many people are hurt/sick?
¿Cuántas personas están heridas/enfermas? [kwán-tas per-son-as es-tán er-ee-das/en-fer-mas]

How old is the patient?
¿Cuántos años tiene el paciente? [kwán-tos an-yos tee-en-eh el pah-see-en-teh]

Is the patient breathing and conscious?
¿El paciente está respirando y está consciente? [el pah-see-en-teh es-tá res-peer-ando ee es-tá kon-see-en-teh]

How far was the fall?
¿Qué tan alto estaba? [keh tan alto es-taba]

What caused the fall/accident?
¿Qué causó la caída o el accidente? [keh kow-só la ka-ee-da o el ax-ee-den-teh]

Is there any serious bleeding?
¿Hay alguien que esté sangrando mucho? [ay al-gee-en keh es-téh san-gran-doh moo-cho]

What part of the body was injured?

¿Qué parte del cuerpo fue herida?
[keh par-te del koo-ehr-poh fweh er-ee-da]

When did the fall/accident happen?
¿Cuándo pasó la caída o el accidente? [kwán-do pa-só la ka-ee-da oh el ax-ee-den-teh]

Responses:

Yes I'm with the patient.
Sí, estoy con el paciente. [see, es-toy kon el pah-see-en-teh]

No, I'm not with the patient.
No, no estoy con el paciente. [no, no es-toy kon pah-see-en-teh]

_____ (two) people are sick/ hurt.
_____ (dos) personas están enfermas/heridas. [dos per-son-as están en-fer-mas/er-ee-das]

The patient is _____ years old.
El paciente tiene _____ años. [el pah-see-en-teh tee-en-eh _____ an-yos]

Yes, the patient is conscious.
Sí, el paciente está consciente. [see el pah-see-en-tehes-tá kon-see-en-teh]

No, the patient is not conscious.
No, el paciente no está consciente. [no el pah-see-en-teh no es-tá kon-see-en-teh]

The patient fell ____ feet/meters.
El paciente cayó a ____ pies/metros de altura. [el pah-see-en-teh kai-ó a ____ pee-es/meh-tros de al-too-ra]

The person injured their arm/leg/head/back/whole body.
La persona se lastimó el brazo/pierna/cabeza/espalda/cuerpo completo. [la per-sona se las-tee-mó el bra-zo/pee-er-na/kah-beh-za/es-pal-da/ku-er-po kom-ple-toh]

The patient is not breathing.
El paciente no está respirando. [el pah-see-en-teh no es-tá res-peer-an-doh]

The patient does not have a pulse.
El paciente no tiene pulso. [el pah-see-en-teh no tee-en-eh pool-so]

The patient was assaulted.
El paciente fue asaltado(a) [el pah-see-en-teh fue ah-sal-tah-doh(a)]

The patient was in a car/motorcycle/bike accident.
El paciente estuvo en un accidente automovilístico. [elpah-see-en-teh es-too-boh en un ax-ee-den-teh auto-mo-bil-ee-stee-koh]

POLICE

Questions:

Are you at the location now?
> **¿Estás en el domicilio en este momento?** [es-tás en el dom-ee-see-lee-oh en es-te mo-men-toh]

When did this happen?
> **¿Cuándo pasó esto?** [kwán-doh pa-só es-toh]

Does the person appear to have a weapon?
> **¿La persona tenía un arma?** [la per-sona ten-ee-ah un ar-mah]

Can you describe what is happening?
> **¿Puedes describir qué está pasando?** [pwe-des des-creeb-eer keh es-tá pas-an-doh]

Can you give me a description of the person?
> **¿Me puedes dar una descripción de la persona?** [meh pue-des dar una des-kreep-see-ón de la per-son-ah]

Where is the person now?
> **¿Dónde está la persona ahora?** [dón-de es-tah la per-son-ah ah-or-ah]

Responses:

Yes, I'm at the location right now.
Sí, actualmente estoy en el domicilio. [see, ak-tu-al-men-teh es-toy en el dom-ee-see-lee-oh]

No, I am not at the location right now.
No, no estoy en el domicilio en este momento. [no, no es-toy en el dom-ee-see-lee-oh en es-te mo-men-toh]

Yes, the person has a gun/knife/sharp object.
Sí, la persona tiene un arma/cuchillo/objeto filoso. [see, la-per-son-ah tee-en-eh un ar-mah/ku-chee-oh/ob-hek-to fil-oh-so]

No, the person does not have a weapon.
No, la persona no tiene un arma. [no, la per-son-ah no tee-en-eh un ar-mah]

There is a fight.
Hay una pelea. [ay una pe-leh-ah]

Someone is trying to hurt me.
Alguien está intentando herirme. [al-gee-en es-tá een-ten-tando er-eer-meh]

Someone is trying to break into my house.
Alguien está intentando entrar a mi casa. [al-gee-en es-tá een-ten-tahn-doh en-trar a mee ka-sah]

Someone just hurt me.
Alguien me acaba de lastimar. [al-gee-en meh ah-kah-bah de last-ee-mar]
I am going to kill myself/someone.
Me voy a matar. Mataré a alguien. [meh boy a ma-tar. mat-ar-éh a al-gee-en]
Someone stole my wallet/car/phone/purse.
Alguien robó mi cartera/carro/teléfono/bolsa. [al-gee-en ro-bó mee kar-tera/karr-ro/tel-éh-fo-no/bol-sah]

The person is/has - **La persona es/tiene** [la per-son-ah es/tee-en-eh]

Male/Female/Unidentifiable.
Mujer/Hombre/Inidentificable. [moo-her/om-breh/een-ee-den-tee-fee-ka-bleh]
Short/tall.
Bajo/alto. [ba-ho/al-toh]
Heavy/thin.
Robusto/flaco. [ro-boos-toh/fla-ko]
Has black/brown/red/blonde hair.
Tiene pelo negro/café/rojo/claro. [tee-en-eh peh-lo neg-roh/ka-féh/ro-ho/kla-ro]
Is bald.
Es calvo. [es kal-bo]
Tattoos on their face/neck/arm/leg/body.

Tiene tatuajes en su cara/cuello/pierna/cuerpo. [tee-en-es tah-too-ah-hes en su ka-ra/ku-eh-yo/pee-er-nah/ku-er-po]

Wearing a jacket/pants/shorts/shirt/shoes/boots.

Llevaba una chaqueta/pantalones/zapatos/botas. [ye-bah-bah una cha-ke-ta/pan-tah-lon-es/za-pah-tos/bo-tas]

The person has left the scene.

La persona ya se ha ido del lugar. [la per-son-ah ya se ah ee-doh del loo-gar]

The person is still here.

La persona todavía está aquí. [la per-son-ah to-da-bee-ah es-tá ah-key]

The person left in a_____ vehicle.

La persona se fue en un vehículo _____. [la per-son-ah se fwe en un beh-hee-koo-loh]

Color- black, brown, grey, white, red. /

Color negro, café, gris, blanco, rojo, azul. [ko-lor neg-roh, ka-féh, grees, blan-ko ro-ho, ah-zool]

Year- old/new

Año - viejo/reciente. [an-yo - bee-eh-ho/re-see-en-teh]

Model (of vehicle)

Modelo (de vehículo) [mo-deh-lo (de beh-hee-koo-loh)]

License plate state and number.
Número de placa _____ y estado _____ [noo-mer-oh de pla-ka____ ee es-ta-doh]

FIRE

Questions:

Do you see flames?
> **¿Ves flamas?** [bes flah-mas]

Do you see smoke?
> **¿Ves humo?** [bes oo-moh]

How many floors are in the building?
> **¿Cuántos pisos hay en el edificio?** [kwán-tos pee-sos ay en el eh-dee-fee-see-oh]

Is anyone in the building?
> **¿Hay alguien en el edificio?** [ay al-gee-en en el eh-dee-fee-see-oh]

Responses:

There is a fire.
> **Hay un incendio.** [ay un in-sen-dee-oh]

Yes, there is smoke.
> **Sí, hay humo.** [see, ay oo-moh]

No, there is no smoke.
> **No, no hay humo.** [no, no ay oo-moh]

Yes, I see flames.
> **Sí, veo flamas.** [see, be-oh flah-mas]

No, I do not see flames.
> **No, no veo flamas.** [no, no be-oh flah-mas]

The fire is in a house/apartment/building.

El incendio está en una casa/apartamento/edificio. [el in-sen-dee-od es-tá en una ka-sah/ap-ar-ta-men-to/eh-dee-fee-see-oh]

The building has _____ stories/floors.
El edificio tiene _____ pisos. [el eh-dee-fee-see-oh tee-en-eh _____ pee-sos]

Yes, there are people in the building.
Sí, hay gente en el edificio. [see, ay hen-teh en el eh-dee-fee-see-oh]

I don't know if there are people in the building.
No sé si haya gente en el edificio. [no seh see aya hen-teh en el eh-dee-fee-see-oh]

OTHER

Help is on the way.
> **La ayuda va en camino.** [la ay-oo-dah va en kam-een-oh]

Please do not hang up the phone.
> **Por favor no cuelgues el teléfono.** [por fah-vor no ku-el-ges el tel-éh-fono]

Are you there still?
> **¿Todavía estás ahí?** [to-da-bee-ah es-tas ah-ee]

Remain calm.
> **Guarda la calma.** [gwar-da la kal-mah]

Help will be there soon.
> **La ayuda estará ahí pronto.** [la ay-oo-dah es-tar-áh ah-ee pron-toh]

Conclusion: Dispatch

It is important for emergency dispatchers to have excellent verbal communication skills, as they are the first ones to respond to an emergency but cannot use their own eyes to assess a situation. The goal of *Part 5: Dispatch* is to provide emergency dispatchers the necessarily basic knowledge of the Spanish language that will help facilitate the communication process.

Closing Comments

Spanish for Emergency Medical Services was written with the intention of providing a quality resource specifically designed for Paramedics, EMTs, Dispatchers, and other medical professionals. *Part 1: Spanish Language Basics* and *Part 2: Greetings & Commonly Used Language* provide information for a strong base knowledge of the Spanish language. The rest of the book focuses on teaching the necessary language and vocabulary that is most useful for the healthcare provider and emergency responder. You should now have the knowledge and ability to effectively communicate with patients using medical Spanish.

Successfully learning another language involves more than just learning the written form. It is imperative that listening and speaking skills are as equally developed as reading and writing skills. The best way to practice speaking and listening comprehension skills is to practice with another person. Otherwise, use a simple search on the internet for videos, articles, books, and more that are easy to find. Use resources that are best for your learning style.

Always continue learning.

Thank you!

www.ingramcontent.com/pod-product-compliance
Lightning Source LLC
Chambersburg PA
CBHW070634220526
45466CB00001B/176